DIAGNOSING THE DIAGNOSTIC AND STATISTICAL MANUAL OF MENTAL DISORDERS

DIAGNOSING THE DIAGNOSTIC AND STATISTICAL MANUAL OF MENTAL DISORDERS

Rachel Cooper

KARNAC

First published in 2014 by
Karnac Books Ltd
118 Finchley Road
London NW3 5HT

Copyright © 2014 by Rachel Cooper

The right of Rachel Cooper to be identified as the author of this work has been asserted in accordance with §§ 77 and 78 of the Copyright Design and Patents Act 1988.

All rights reserved. No part of this publication may be reproduced, stored in a retrieval system, or transmitted, in any form or by any means, electronic, mechanical, photocopying, recording, or otherwise, without the prior written permission of the publisher.

British Library Cataloguing in Publication Data

A C.I.P. for this book is available from the British Library

ISBN-13: 978-1-85575-825-4

Typeset by V Publishing Solutions Pvt Ltd., Chennai, India

Printed in Great Britain

www.karnacbooks.com

CONTENTS

ACKNOWLEDGEMENTS   vii

ABOUT THE AUTHOR   viii

INTRODUCING THE DSM   ix

CHAPTER ONE
DSM-5: an overview of changes   1

CHAPTER TWO
Controversies of process: the DSM
    and the pharmaceutical industry   13

CHAPTER THREE
Controversies of process: transparency
    and patient involvement   21

CHAPTER FOUR
Issues of content: the birth of a new
    diagnosis—hoarding disorder   31

CHAPTER FIVE
Issues of content: the changing limits of autistic
    spectrum disorders   40

CHAPTER SIX
The field trials: DSM-5 and the new crisis
    of reliability   49

CHAPTER SEVEN
The future   56

REFERENCES   62

INDEX   75

ACKNOWLEDGEMENTS

Many people have helped me in writing this book. I owe particular thanks to the publishers, Karnac, who suggested the project.

The American Psychiatric Association gave me access to its archives relating to the DSM-III and DSM-IV. Gary McMillan, archivist at the American Psychiatric Association, was generous both with muscle and brainpower. He shifted many boxes of files and helped me make sense of their contents.

The British Academy funded this research. A mid-career fellowship paid for my visit to the archives, and also funded my study leave while this book was written.

Rowan Hildebrand-Chupp introduced me to the wonders of The Wayback Machine, an internet archive site. Victoria Allison-Bolger, Sam Fellowes, Sara Mellen and Mariana Salcedo read drafts and made many helpful comments. I also owe thanks to my partner, Trevor Steele, who did more than his fair share of childcare and washing-up while I finished this book. Finally, I should like to thank Fran Shall, who copy-edited the text.

ABOUT THE AUTHOR

Rachel Cooper studied for her PhD in history and philosophy of science at Cambridge University and is currently a senior lecturer in philosophy at Lancaster University, UK. She works mainly on conceptual problems around the classification of mental disorders. Her previous publications include *Classifying Madness* (Springer, 2005) and *Psychiatry and the Philosophy of Science* (Acumen, 2007).

INTRODUCING THE DSM

This is a short book about a long book. The long book is the *Diagnostic and Statistical Manual of Mental Disorders*, more commonly known as the DSM. The DSM aims to list and describe all psychiatric disorders, focusing on those seen relatively often in the United States. It is published by the American Psychiatric Association (APA), and undergoes a major revision every fifteen years or so. The latest version, the DSM-5, was published in May 2013. This book concentrates on issues more or less specifically relating to this edition.

The DSM provides a set of diagnostic criteria for each disorder. This lists the symptoms that must be present before the disorder can be diagnosed. Disorder 303.00 alcohol intoxication, for example, is to be used when a certain number of characteristic symptoms (slurred speech, unsteady gait, impairment in attention or memory, and so on) follow "recent ingestion of alcohol". For 300.4 persistent depressive disorder symptoms can include problems with appetite and sleep, fatigue, low self-esteem, poor concentration, and feelings of hopelessness. Notably, the symptom lists often require only that a patient display some subset of a longer list (three from five, say). As a consequence, patients with the same diagnosis may have rather different symptoms. In addition to the symptom list, many diagnostic criteria also include an age restriction (some diagnoses are for children, others for adults), a duration requirement (symptoms must often be present for some minimum time), and various exclusion criteria (commonly, symptoms must not be caused by a somatic medical disorder). Frequently, it is also required that symptoms must cause "clinically significant" distress or impairment before a diagnosis can be given. For each disorder the accompanying text gives additional information, and describes prevalence, sex differences, cultural variations, and so on.

Internationally, the DSM is central to mental health research. Most papers published in psychiatric journals refer to the DSM; its categories are almost universally employed to select subject populations for study. Clinical trials seek to show that a drug is a useful treatment for this or that DSM category. Worldwide, textbooks for mental health professionals tend to be structured around DSM categories. The DSM also plays an important cultural role in delimiting the boundaries of mental disorder, and conversely of normality. Discussions of mental health, whether in popular magazines, on TV, or on the web, often refer to DSM diagnostic categories. In the US, the DSM also takes on crucial economic importance; before insurers will pay for mental health treatment, a DSM code is commonly required.

In addition to the DSM, there is also another important classification of mental disorders. The World Health Organisation (WHO) publishes the *International Classification of Diseases* (ICD), which supplies codes for official health statistics for the whole of medicine. The ICD includes a chapter dedicated to "Mental and Behavioural Disorders". However, at present the ICD and DSM can scarcely count as distinct classifications of mental disorders. Over the last few decades, the APA and the WHO have sought to align the DSM and ICD, with the result that the two are now very similar (First, 2009).[1] The mental disorders section of the forthcoming ICD-11 is expected to be much the same as the DSM-5.

These days, the DSM is big, expensive, influential, and widely used, but this wasn't always so. The first DSM, published in 1952, was designed specifically to enable the collection of statistics on hospital inpatients. It was slim, cheap, and little read. The DSM-II published in 1968 was slightly bigger but only marginally more influential. Not until the third edition in 1980 did the DSM take more or less its current form, and really start to matter. From then on each new edition—DSM-III-R in 1987, DSM-IV in 1994, DSM-IV-TR in 2000 (with the "R" standing for "revision" and the "TR" for "text revision")—got bigger, and pricier, and further helped to consolidate the system's position as the premier classification of mental disorders.

Nowadays, revising the DSM is a major undertaking. Work on producing the DSM-5 began in earnest in 2006 and has cost about $25 million (Frances, 2013, p. 175). As publisher of the DSM, the APA controls the process by which it is revised. A task force of about thirty, chaired by David Kupfer and Darrel Regier, oversaw the project. Each section of the manual—mood disorders, childhood disorders, and so on—was reviewed by an associated work group of about ten experts. Members of the work groups reviewed the literature published since DSM-IV and considered where the classification might be in need of updating. They presented their ideas in published papers and at conferences to gather feedback. Draft proposals for changes to the DSM diagnostic criteria were posted online, and anyone who wanted was able to email their comments to the APA. Some of the new diagnostic criteria sets were tested in field trials, where clinicians used the draft criteria to check that they could be understood and used in practice. Finally, before publication, the DSM had to be voted through by the various committees of the APA.

That, at least, is the official story of the process by which the DSM was revised. The official story is true, but it's not the whole truth. Behind the scenes, other forces were also at work. The DSM matters and so many are motivated to seek to influence it. Patients and mental health professionals lobby to try to ensure that the DSM reflects their interests. Generally such lobbying extends beyond the life of a single edition of the DSM. Revising the DSM now takes so long that work on revision is almost constant; as soon as one edition goes to press, discussion on how it should be revised begins. With each revision, diagnoses can be included or excluded, expanded or restricted. Interested groups must thus maintain pressure to ensure that their interests are protected, and lobbying activities can go on for decades: to get a single edition of the DSM as one desires is only to win a battle—winning the war requires longer-term effort.

Some want "their" condition to be included. The most common reason for wanting to be "in" is that diagnosis frequently acts to unlock funding for treatment or services. As documented by Allan Young in *The Harmony of Illusions* (1997), lobbying by well-organised groups of traumatised Vietnam veterans, and their therapists, helped ensure that post-traumatic stress disorder was included in the DSM-III in 1980. The inclusion of this combat-related diagnosis in the DSM was crucial for gaining treatment funding from the Veterans Health Administration. Groups representing adults with attention deficit/hyperactivity disorder (Ramsay & Waite, no date), and family therapists who treat relational disorders (Kaslow, 1993; Denton, 2007), have also wanted greater visibility for "their" conditions in the DSM. Others want to be out of the classification. Many would prefer to be given a somatic medical diagnosis, and avoid the stigma of having a psychiatric disorder. Groups concerned with ME/chronic fatigue syndrome have been especially active in this regard (McCleary, 2010). At various points, groups have also lobbied for stuttering (*Psychiatric News*, 1980), Tourette's syndrome (Kushner, 1999, 2004), and transsexualism (Knudson, De Cuypere, & Bockting, 2010), to be regarded as physical diagnoses. Others protest the notion that they suffer from a disorder of any kind. Homosexuality is, of course, the classic example of a condition once included in the DSM and now regarded as normal (Bayer, 1981). Some transsexual groups currently lobby to be regarded as non-disordered (Knudson, De Cuypere, & Bockting, 2010). Others who have lobbied to be seen as normal include groups representing the bereaved (Kluger, Cacciatore, & Montgomery, 2012), and women who experience mood fluctuations with their menstrual cycle (Caplan, 1995, ch. 5).

Pharmaceutical companies also have interests in the DSM. When a diagnostic category comes to be included in the DSM, or existing categories are expanded, multimillion-dollar markets for drugs are created. Industry has the influence and money to shape psychiatric opinion to promote its concerns. Researchers with economically useful ideas are supported, and are provided with funding for studies, research centres, travel to conferences, and so on. The end result is that ideas that are useful to industry come to be better known than those that are not. The consensus of experts can thus come to reflect industry interests, and, in due course, the consensus of experts also comes to be reflected in the DSM.

At the time of writing, the DSM-5 has only just been published. This book is very much a preliminary assessment of its contents and the processes via which it was revised. For the time being, much of the nitty-gritty regarding the development of the DSM-5 remains known only to APA committee members, and they have been bound to secrecy (Board of Trustees, 2007). Still, there is every reason to think the processes by which the DSM-5 has been developed will have been similar to those used in earlier revisions. As part of the research for this book, I visited the archives of the APA to review documents relating to the construction of the DSM-III, III-R, and DSM-IV (documents relating to the DSM-5 will not be made available to researchers for some time). What I saw in the archives, especially in relation to the later editions, was impressive. The files relating to the DSM-IV in particular are huge. There are boxes full of materials—offprints of works relating to psychiatric classification, literature reviews produced for the committees considering changes, data related to field trials, reanalyses of existing relevant data sets, the minutes of many meetings, and files and files of letters and petitions from individuals and lobby groups seeking to influence the process. Assuming the work associated with the DSM-5 was similar to that associated with the DSM-IV, the committees will have worked very hard, they will have reviewed massive literatures, they will have consulted widely; for the most part they will have done their best. Despite this work, as I will explain in the rest of this book, I think that problems with the DSM remain.

The DSM is extremely controversial, and only some issues will be dealt with here. Some challenge the very idea of classifying mental distress. Outside the counselling offices at my university, a sign bears the slogan "Labels are for jars, not people"—a slogan also used in demonstrations against the DSM at the APA annual meeting in 2012 (Davies, 2012). The concerns of those who think that classifying mental distress does more harm than good should be taken seriously—but not here.[2] In this book I focus on the more local concerns of those who are happy enough with the general idea of psychiatric classification, but who wonder whether the DSM-5 classifies the right people in the right way.

In greater detail, Chapter One presents an overview of the main changes between the DSM-5 and its predecessors. Chapters Two and Three look at possible worries about the process by which the DSM-5 was constructed. Chapter Two focuses on potential conflicts of interest produced by links between the DSM-5 and the pharmaceutical industry. Chapter Three examines controversies about transparency, and in particular looks at the (limited) role that patient groups have played in the construction of the DSM-5. Chapters Four and Five focus on controversies about disorders added to and removed from the DSM. Chapter Four looks at hoarding disorder, a disorder new to the DSM-5, and uses this as a case study for exploring concerns that surround the expansion of the psychiatric domain. Chapter Five focuses on the most prominent removal from the classification, Asperger's disorder, which has been removed as a standalone diagnosis and is now subsumed into autistic spectrum disorder. Chapter Six looks at the field trials, which offer the first clues as to how the new classification may operate in practice, and discusses problems with the reliability of the newly proposed categories. Chapter Seven, the final chapter, considers the future. The chapters are written to be self-standing, and can be read in any order.

Before we begin, a note regarding terminology is needed. In writing about mental health what one calls those who are diagnosed has become a politicised issue. To caricature, the reactionary term is "patient", the politically correct term "user" or "client", the radical term "survivor". I find there is no ideal term, and will resort to "patient", though I consider myself no reactionary. I reject "survivor", short for "psychiatric system survivor", as I find it too angry. It is true that many find the mental health care that they receive to be unhelpful, but others find it useful. I also dislike "client" and "user". I worry that such terms serve to obscure the political and economic context in which mental health services are provided. In most client-professional relationships, the client pays the professional, who acts in the client's interests. Many mental health services do not fit this model; some mental health care is coercive, and much is neither funded nor controlled by those who are treated. Given that many mental health "clients" are only "clients" in an Orwellian sense, I prefer the term "patient".

As this book is about the DSM it discusses DSM diagnostic criteria frequently. To avoid cluttering the text, where I discuss DSM diagnostic criteria I have not supplied page references. All editions of the DSM are well organised and the relevant diagnostic criteria are easy to find.

Notes

1. First documents the many small differences between DSM-IV and ICD-10. The aim of his paper is to draw attention to the current differences between the systems, which he views as an impediment to research. However, despite the many small differences, overall the two systems are very similar.
2. In Cooper (2012) I begin to address these broader issues.

CHAPTER ONE

DSM-5: an overview of changes

These days, as soon as one edition of the DSM goes to press, work on the next begins. The revision process that culminated in the publication of DSM-5 thus started long ago; with pipe dreams that finally came to nothing. An early publication, *A Research Agenda for DSM-V* (the Latin numerals only changed later) set out the ambitions (Kupfer, First, & Regier, 2002). *A Research Agenda for DSM-V* is an extraordinary document. The book doesn't consist of plans for DSM-5 but rather of plans for plans; a series of "white papers" outline research priorities in various areas relevant to psychiatric classification. It is a testament to the phenomenal success of the DSM that such a book should be published, and not only published but published in paperback; research *proposals* related to psychiatric classification now find a mass readership. The very term "white paper", used by the editors to describe the chapters, is more normally associated with plans produced by the offices of nation states. Though partly bluster, such self-importance is basically justified. Given that millions of people worldwide suffer from mental disorders, and that the DSM diagnosis someone receives can determine whether and how they are treated, changes to the DSM can potentially affect the lives of as many people as changes in the policies of most countries.

In retrospect perhaps unwisely, *A Research Agenda for DSM-V* begins by detailing problems with the DSM series to date. The DSM-III, published in 1980, sought to be a purely descriptive classification that made no use of unproven theoretical assumptions (APA, 1980, pp. 6–8). At the time, psychoanalysis remained an important perspective in US psychiatry, and psychoanalytically and biologically inclined psychiatrists could reach agreement on little. It was hoped that producing a theory-free classification would make the DSM acceptable to mental health professionals working within different theoretical frameworks. A key theme of *A Research Agenda for DSM-V* is that the descriptive syndromes included in the DSM have now become so embedded in psychiatric research as to be potentially problematic. It increasingly seems likely that some theoretically interesting populations do not map on to DSM categories, and such groups are currently under-researched. If, for example, some sub-group of those with a particular DSM diagnosis share a genetic abnormality, or a drug can help a population that cuts across current categories, this is likely to be missed by current research programmes. Unfortunately, while *A Research Agenda for DSM-V* is clear that research based on DSM-IV-like categories might well make little progress, it is less clear about what the DSM-5 should offer instead, opining only that some "as yet unknown paradigm shift may need to occur" (Kupfer, First, & Regier, 2002, p. xix). While the chapters of *A Research Agenda for DSM-V* boast about the great advances being made in areas such as neuroscience, developmental science, and cross-cultural studies, each also makes it clear that robust findings that might support a fundamentally different approach to psychiatric classification are a long way off.

In the event, between the publication of *A Research Agenda for DSM-V* (2002) and the publication of DSM-5 (2013) the APA did not develop a new paradigm for psychiatric classification.

In place of a paradigm shift, the DSM-5 offers a chapter reorganisation. In a *Research Agenda for DSM-V* there is much talk of moving towards more dimensional approaches to classifying psychopathology. In the end, efforts to construct a dimensional system failed, but the new organisation of disorders in the DSM-5 is supposed to hint at a more dimensional approach. Disorders that are thought to have a similar origin are now placed together in the classification. This organisation is supposed to be "a bridge to new diagnostic approaches" (APA, 2013, p. 13). The idea is that placing disorders thought similar adjacent to each other will help emphasise the commonalities that run across the diagnostic categories. The categories will thus seem less categorical than under previous organisations, and the APA hopes that this will encourage "broad investigations within the proposed chapters and across adjacent chapters" (APA, 2013, p. 13).

As one might guess from the fact that an anticipated paradigm shift became a chapter reorganisation, the DSM-5 is conservative in outlook. When considering changes to the diagnostic criteria, I shall generally compare the DSM-IV (1994) and the DSM-5. The DSM-IV-TR (2000) was only a "text revision", that is the sets of diagnostic criteria remained the same as in the DSM-IV (with a very few exceptions), and only the accompanying text was revised. Changes in the sets of diagnostic criteria between the DSM-IV and DSM-5 are modest. A few new disorders have been included; a few have been removed. Some diagnostic criteria have changed. One of the issues this book will explore is how it is that making revisions to the DSM has become so very difficult that conservatism tends to prevail. I will also show how it is that each and every small change can matter. When it comes to classification the devil is in the details.

The most controversial changes to the DSM concern possible expansion of the classification. When a new diagnosis comes to be included in the DSM, or an old category is expanded, more people come to be thought of as suffering from mental disorder. The effects of this are multiple, and not all are benign. As Peter Conrad (2007) and other medical sociologists have done so much to show, with diagnosis, the ways in which patients, and others, think about a problem shifts. Diagnosis suggests that the source of a problem should be located within an individual, and indicates that professional medical help is likely to be required. Simultaneously, diagnosis tends to remove an issue from the political or ethical domain. To take an example, consider the effects of the diagnosis of attention deficit/hyperactivity disorder (ADHD). Prior to the omnipresence of ADHD diagnoses, one could imagine many different explanations for the activity of disruptive children. Maybe the teachers are boring? Maybe young children are naturally ill suited to spending days cooped up studying maths? Maybe the problem is simple naughtiness? Maybe contemporary parenting styles are somehow inadequate? Diagnosis with ADHD acts to push these competing explanations to one side. The education system, parents, and the children themselves tend to be absolved from blame. Instead the cause of the disruption is located inside the children's brains, and the remedy frequently proposed is drug treatment.

Some difficulties are caused by problems inside brains, drugs sometimes work, and diagnosis can sometimes be useful. But it is important to remember that diagnosis also produces harm. Not only does an emphasis on medical interventions distract attention from political, economic, and moral changes that might produce preferable results, but also drugs can be overused and have side effects, and stigma and self-stigmatisation can reduce the life opportunities for the diagnosed. As medicalisation has such effects, no expansion of the domain of mental disorder should pass unexamined.

Inclusions to the DSM come in different grades. Most straightforwardly, some new additions make it into the manual proper. These disorders have their own numerical codes and sets of diagnostic criteria and are "fully legitimate" diagnoses.

Other additions have a less clear status. Since DSM-III-R, the DSM has included an appendix listing "Conditions for further study". Conditions in the appendix lack numerical codes, but do have sets of diagnostic criteria. The appendix acts as a halfway house for conditions not yet seen to be fully legitimate for inclusion in the main manual. In the DSM-5, a note states these diagnoses are considered appropriate for research, but not for clinical practice.

There are also some diagnoses that are mentioned in the text of the DSM but that have no accompanying diagnostic criteria sets. The DSM is littered with "ragbag" codes for "other" disorders, for example "other specified anxiety disorder", "other specified feeding or eating disorder". These are provided for patients who the clinician considers to suffer from a disorder of some particular genus but who fail to meet the criteria for any specific coded diagnosis. Sometimes new disorders first make it into the DSM through being listed in the text of the DSM as possible "other" disorders that might appropriately fall under these ragbag codes. For example, restless legs syndrome has been included as a distinct codeable condition for the first time in DSM-5, but was previously described in the text of the DSM-IV as an example of dyssomnia not otherwise specified.

With the DSM-5, conditions that have been introduced to the main body of the classification include, perhaps most controversially, disruptive mood dysregulation disorder, for children with persistent irritability and episodes of behavioural dyscontrol. In the US there has recently been a massive increase in the numbers of children being diagnosed with bipolar disorder. Disruptive mood dysregulation disorder is intended as a more accurate label for these children. It will be discussed in greater detail in Chapter Two.

Other additions include social (pragmatic) communication disorder, a developmental disorder characterised by problems with the social use of language (to be discussed in greater detail in Chapter Five). Binge eating disorder has been upgraded from the appendix, and is as it sounds, a diagnosis for people who binge eat. Excoriation (skin picking) disorder is a new diagnosis, for people who repeatedly pick their skin. In addition to restless legs, rapid eye movement sleep behaviour disorder is another sleep disorder previously only mentioned in the text but now supplied with diagnostic criteria. Hoarding was previously mentioned in the DSM-IV as a possible symptom of obsessive-compulsive personality disorder but is now seen as characterising a distinct condition. Chapter Four will discuss hoarding disorder in greater detail and examine further how it is that new conditions can come to be included in the DSM.

Premenstrual dysphoric disorder, a mood disorder related to the menstrual period (upgraded from the appendix), is a further notable addition. During the construction of the DSM-III, III-R, and DSM-IV this disorder (and its ancestors with different names) was one of the most controversial suggestions for inclusion (for a history of these debates see Caplan, 1995). Then, massive protests by feminists, who feared that it would pathologise normal changes in mood associated with the menstrual period, blocked its inclusion in the main classification. The APA archives contain folders and folders of protest letters. This time round, the upgrading of the disorder to the main body of the classification has passed with little comment.[1]

Amongst new conditions included in the appendix the most controversial are attenuated psychosis syndrome and internet use gaming disorder. Attenuated psychosis syndrome is conceptualised as a condition characterising adolescents at increased risk of developing schizophrenia. Critics worry that this diagnosis may lead to the stigmatisation and over-treatment of peculiar teenagers (Moran, 2009). Internet use gaming disorder concerns some who see it as opening the door to a proliferation of other, behaviour-related "addictions" (sex addiction, exercise addiction, etc.) (Frances, 2013, pp. 188–192).

The domain of psychiatry can also expand as a result of changes to the sets of diagnostic criteria for existing diagnoses. In the DSM-5 numerous small changes, of which I will discuss only a few, may be expected to result in more people being diagnosed with particular conditions. For example, the diagnostic criteria for ADHD have changed to make it easier for adults to receive the diagnosis. Previously symptoms had to have their onset prior to age seven, now the age threshold has been increased to twelve, and the number of symptoms that adults require for diagnosis has also been reduced. In DSM-IV bulimia nervosa and binge eating required binges twice a week for three months, now binges need occur only once a week.

Amongst the most controversial changes to the diagnostic criteria has been the removal of the "grief exclusion" in major depressive disorder (Friedman, 2012; *Lancet*, 2012). Symptoms of bereavement can be similar to those of depression. In DSM-IV, depression could not be diagnosed in recently bereaved people (unless the symptoms were very severe or lasted longer than two months). In DSM-5 the grief exclusion has been removed, although a footnote, added in response to protests, gives guidance as to how a clinician can distinguish between grief and a major depressive episode, and seeks to ensure that only some bereaved people will be diagnosed as depressed.

Most of the changes to diagnostic criteria are carefully considered by the relevant committees (though they may well remain controversial), but on occasion diagnostic expansion occurs by mistake. In *The Book of Woe* (2013), Gary Greenberg interviews Allen Frances, who was chairperson for the DSM-IV and DSM-IV-TR. Frances is now haunted by some of the accidental consequences of the revisions he oversaw. Paraphilias (sexual perversions) were amongst a handful of disorders where diagnostic criteria were changed between DSM-IV and DSM-IV-TR. The result was "one royal fuckup" (to quote Frances) (Greenberg, 2013, p. 233). In

DSM-IV, paraphilias could only be diagnosed if the patient experienced "clinically significant distress or impairment in social, occupational, or other important areas of functioning". Critics became concerned that, say, paedophilia could not be diagnosed in those who were quite happy with their desires and behaviour. In response, the diagnostic criteria were changed, and in DSM-IV-TR many paraphilias could be diagnosed so long as someone had "acted on these urges or is markedly distressed by them". The unintended consequence is that under DSM-IV-TR those who commit sex crimes may meet the diagnostic criteria for a paraphilia by virtue of their crime alone. This goes against traditional psychiatric thinking (and the intentions of the DSM committees) which holds that the majority of sex offenders do not suffer from a mental disorder but are simply criminals. In the context of the US legal system the mistake takes on added significance, as the sexually violent predator laws in many states mean that offenders with a paraphilia diagnosis can be detained indefinitely. On reflection, Frances believes the problems stem from the fact that the diagnostic criteria in DSM-IV-TR contain an "or" instead of an "and". If diagnosis with a paraphilia had required "fantasies, urges, *and* behaviours" rather than "fantasies, urges, *or* behaviours" then many fewer people would be diagnosable.

The DSM-5 may well also contain mistakes that will lead to the incidence of diagnoses changing in unexpected ways, though it is in the nature of such errors that they tend to become obvious only after a new edition has been in use for some years. One change in the DSM-5 that may have unintended consequences has occurred in the criteria for phobias. Previously patients had to recognise their fears as unreasonable, but now the fear merely has to be judged by the clinician to be out of proportion. This change has been introduced as many older adults who develop intense fears, say of falling, perceive their fears to be reasonable (LeBeau et al., 2010). However, potentially, this change has the consequence that those who develop rational fears on the basis of information that the diagnosing clinician lacks may be diagnosed. Suppose, for example, that I have unusual expertise: I study data about air traffic control systems. Based on my work, I come to believe the system is near collapse. I develop rational fears about plane crashes. Under the DSM-IV I did not have a phobia, as I would not have considered my fears unreasonable, but under DSM-5, if my clinician (who we will suppose knows nothing of these matters) judges my fear as being out of proportion, I can receive a diagnosis.

Some key critics of the DSM-5 worry that it will expand the domain of psychiatry and pathologise much normal behaviour. Allen Frances believes that work now needs to be done to "save normal" (Frances, 2013). Some of the revisions to the DSM-5 will certainly act to increase the rates of diagnosis of some disorders. But while the DSM-5 extends the reach of psychiatry in some directions, it reduces it in others. Some diagnoses have been removed from the classification, and some diagnostic criteria have been tightened.

The most controversial exclusion from DSM-5 is Asperger's disorder, which is now subsumed within autistic spectrum disorder. The rise and fall of Asperger's has been rapid. Asperger's first made it into the DSM only with DSM-IV in 1994, and even then its inclusion wasn't agreed until late on in the revision process (the 1993 draft notes that it might be placed in the appendix (APA, 1993, p. E.7)). When included, Asperger's was described as a disorder "not familiar to most American psychiatrists" (Volkmar et al., 1994, p. 1362). Since inclusion, Asperger's has come to be a commonly made diagnosis. For many, a diagnosis of Asperger's has ensured the supply of various services and benefits. For some, the diagnosis of Asperger's has also enabled the development of an "aspie" culture and identity.[2] The net result is that quite a lot of people diagnosed with Asperger's like having their diagnosis and fear the consequences of it being subsumed within autistic spectrum disorder. Debates about the removal of Asperger's disorder will be addressed in greater detail in Chapter Five.

The intention is that most of those who would have received a DSM-IV diagnosis of Asperger's disorder will be eligible for a DSM-5 diagnosis of autistic spectrum disorder (although as we shall see in Chapter Five whether this will be the case is contested). Some of the other DSM-IV disorders related to autism have been more thoroughly deleted. In DSM-IV childhood disintegrative disorder could be diagnosed in children who initially developed normally but who then regressed into an autism-like state prior to age ten. In DSM-5, there is no obvious diagnosis for any patients who develop an autism-like disorder in later childhood; childhood disintegrative disorder has disappeared, and a diagnosis of autistic spectrum disorder requires that symptoms be present in the "early developmental period". Whether these changes will affect anyone is unclear. Childhood disintegrative disorder was rarely diagnosed, and cases with late onset were rarely reported (Volkmar, 1992).

Another DSM-IV diagnosis that has been removed is sexual aversion disorder, for people who are averse to sex. Again, this was a rarely used diagnosis. Some who would have been diagnosed with sexual aversion disorder under DSM-IV will now meet criteria for a specific phobia (of sex) under DSM-5.

As well as some diagnoses having been removed, changes to diagnostic criteria mean that quite a few diagnoses will now be harder to make. In particular, criteria for many of the sexual disorders and sleep-wake disorders have been tightened. In DSM-IV the diagnostic criteria for sexual disorders (erectile disorder, female orgasmic disorder, etc.) gave no guidance as to how long the problem needed to have persisted prior to diagnosis. Now six months is required. Previously it was sufficient for diagnosis that the condition cause "interpersonal difficulty" (e.g., it upset one's partner). Now the condition must cause distress "in the individual". In the sleep-wake disorders, in many cases the duration and frequency of required symptoms has increased, and it is now made clearer that the problems can't simply be produced by an unfavourable environment (e.g., for insomnia disorder a criterion has been added that the sleep difficulty must persist despite opportunity for sleep). Other diagnoses that have been tightened include body dysmorphic disorder (a disorder in which someone falsely comes to believe that they have a bodily defect) where a new criterion requires that the "individual engages in repetitive behaviours (e.g., mirror checking, reassurance seeking) or mental acts (e.g., comparing with others) in response to concerns", and dissociative identity disorder (previously multiple personality disorder) which newly requires that the patient suffer clinically significant distress or impairment.

When a diagnosis is removed, or criteria are tightened, it is still technically possible for patients who would previously have received the diagnosis to be given one of the ragbag "other" disorder codes. This said, often the bureaucratic systems under which clinical care operates make the use of "other" codes problematic or pointless. For example, often the main aim of diagnosis is to justify funding for treatment, but many funders will query "other" codes.

Predicting which changes to the DSM will turn out to be significant is difficult. In research, diagnoses may be made strictly according to DSM criteria, but this may not be the case in clinical practice. Gary Greenberg, who works as a psychotherapist in the US, believes that most of his colleagues are "content to find a label that matches people in some vague way" (2013, p. 253). In his view, "Most clinicians don't care what the DSM's rules are." (2013, p. 68).[3] James Phillips, an American psychiatrist, agrees that "practitioners, if they use the manuals at all, use them in a loose, informal manner and are comfortable ignoring diagnostic criteria" (2010, p. 70). A 2008 study of diagnoses of autistic spectrum disorders backs up these claims. Williams et al. (2008) found that most of the children given diagnoses of Asperger's, for example, did not actually meet DSM-IV diagnostic criteria. As will become clear in the course of this book, the rates with which diagnoses are made depend not only on the contents of the DSM, but also on the economic, cultural, and bureaucratic contexts within which diagnoses are made. This means one can't predict in advance of an edition having been used for some years which changes to the DSM will turn out to matter: while some changes will come to affect the lives of millions, others will pass largely unnoticed.

Notes

1. Caplan published a critical article in the popular magazine, *Ms*, in 2008 but there have been no widespread protests about the promotion of premenstrual dysphoric disorder to the main body of the classification.
2. Note that only some of those diagnosed with Asperger's identify with the label, others dislike it.
3. Note that not even the copy editors read the DSM text thoroughly. In DSM-5, for example, the new disorder of disruptive mood dysregulation disorder is variously described as a diagnosis for children under 18 (on pages 156 and 810) and under 12 (on page 155).

CHAPTER TWO

Controversies of process: the DSM and the pharmaceutical industry

Whenever a new condition is included in the DSM, or diagnostic boundaries are expanded, a new market for drugs is potentially created. The pharmaceutical industry thus has huge amounts at stake when the DSM is revised. Given that the DSM matters to the pharmaceutical companies, and given that these companies are rich and powerful, there is cause to monitor links between the drugs industry, the APA, and the DSM.

Let's start with the money. A substantial proportion of the APA's revenue comes from pharmaceutical companies (in 2005, $18 million of a total revenue of $61, down to about $7 million of $46 million by 2011) (APA, 2005, 2012a, 2012b). This money comes partly from advertising in APA journals, partly from sponsorship of the annual meeting, and partly through grants for "education, advocacy and research" (APA, 2012a). Other medical specialties also have links with the pharmaceutical industry, and concern about potential conflicts of interest has become widespread (Kaplan, 2008). In line with actions taken by the professional bodies of other medical specialties, in recent years the APA has sought to institute a range of measures aimed at reducing and managing conflicts of interest (Kaplan, 2008). By 2009, drug money going into the APA had significantly declined (both as the APA set out to reduce the number of industry sponsored symposia at its meetings and as the economic downturn reduced advertising revenue) (Cassels, 2010). In addition to general concerns about the APA being so heavily reliant on funding from the pharmaceutical industry, there are more specific worries about links between industry and members of the committees revising the DSM. Individual committee members may have links with industry, such as receiving fees for speaking and consulting, receiving research grants, and having company shares. Many worry that such industry ties might influence committee members.

The APA has introduced measures to address potential conflicts of interest affecting the DSM. Members of the DSM-5 task force and work groups were required to disclose links with industry. For the duration of their tenure, committee members were required to limit payments from industry to $10,000 annually and stock in pharmaceutical and allied companies to $50,000 (APA, no date). These restrictions have affected many committee members. Cosgrove and Krimsky (2012) found that based on disclosures posted as of January 2012, "69% of DSM-5 task force members report having ties to industry". Many task force and work group members de-invested to a very great extent in order to be able to contribute towards revising the DSM; the chair of the mood disorders work group, Jan Fawcett, likened the sacrifice involved to a "financial colonoscopy" (Whoriskey, 2012).

It is commendable that the APA has sought to limit conflicts of interest in revising the DSM, but there are reasons to worry that its efforts will be inadequate. The guidelines rely on the idea that committee members who largely forgo industry money for the few years that they serve on a committee will thereby be rendered unbiased. This may not be so. On one model the ties between drugs companies and researchers are not merely ones of straightforward exchange (for example, where a psychiatrist provides advice and receives an agreed amount of cash) but rather industry monies act to build up long-term *gift relationships* with researchers (Mather, 2005). As understood by anthropologists, a gift relationship is created when gifts are given and received over time, and thereby create real but non-explicit obligations for reciprocation in the future. In so far as this is true, although committee members may cut industry links for the duration of their tenure, the relationships between industry and the researchers will not thereby be broken. Industry will expect committee members to reciprocate past gifts, and committee members will expect to once again reap benefits from industry once their tenure is finished. Thus, even though a committee member may cut accountable ties with industry for a few years, the expectations and obligations between company and committee member will persist.

In any case, it is probable that the mechanisms by which pharmaceutical companies may influence the DSM do not depend on any money ever passing into the hands of the APA or those directly responsible for revisions. Industry money can come to influence the DSM via a less direct route. Research, and its dissemination, takes money. Much research into mental health is now industry funded. Industry identifies key psychiatrists who have views that support industry interests. Pharmaceutical company money is used to promote these thinkers' work: their studies are sponsored, funding is made available for them to travel and give talks, and help is provided to write papers. Such support can make a particular view more prominent. Patient groups can also act as important allies. When their views are useful, drug company money can enable patient groups to become more efficient lobbyists for change.[1]

In *The Antidepressant Era* (1997), David Healy shows how the category of depression has come to be split in succeeding editions of the DSM, largely, he thinks, as a result of pressures stemming from the pharmaceutical industry. The motivation for splitting arises as follows. Suppose a new antidepressant is manufactured, but it cannot be shown to be a better treatment than existing drugs. Rather than consigning such a drug to the dustbin, a marketing campaign can come into operation. The drug may be no better than competitors for general treatment, but it may still be sold if it can be argued to have advantages in the treatment of some particular *type* of depression—depression mixed with anxiety, or depression with panic attacks, say. To pursue such a strategy the company needs to make it plausible that the subtype exists, that it is quite prevalent, and that their drug is a good treatment for it. With luck, this may be achieved by the targeted funding of medical research and patient groups. Healy argues that over time, such practices have led to disorders such as panic disorder, obsessive-compulsive disorder, and social anxiety disorder coming to be seen as distinct from depression and included in the DSM.

Turning to the DSM-5, the introduction of the new disorder of disruptive mood dysregulation provides another example where pharmaceutical company money has had an impact on the DSM—although in this case perhaps not in quite the ways the companies intended. Over the last few decades there has been a massive increase in diagnoses of bipolar disorder amongst US children; amongst outpatients there was a fortyfold increase in diagnoses from 1994 to 2003 (Moreno et al., 2007). This has been fired by researchers who think that symptoms of bipolar disorder in children might vary from those seen in adults (Parens & Johnston, 2010). While adults experience periods of depression and mania, which might alternate over a period of months or years, some claim that in children irritability might replace classic mania, and that moods might change in a more rapid cycle (on a timescale of days, or even hours). The widespread acceptance of such views has led to DSM-IV criteria for bipolar disorder being interpreted leniently in the case of children, and to the massive increase in rates of diagnosis.

CONTROVERSIES OF PROCESS: THE PHARMACEUTICAL INDUSTRY 17

The diagnosis of children with bipolar disorder is highly controversial. Diagnosis often, although not always, leads to long-term treatment with a cocktail of drugs that generally includes antipsychotics (Moreno et al., 2007). These drugs can have severe side effects and there has been widespread concern about the consequences of their long-term use in children.

To illustrate how drugs company money helped fuel the epidemic, let's focus on the impact of the work of Joseph Biederman. Biederman is a hugely influential psychiatrist; in 2007 he was ranked the second most cited psychiatrist worldwide, with 217 papers cited a total of 6,030 times over the past ten years (In-cites, 2007). His research centre is the Johnson and Johnson Centre for Paediatric Psychopathology at Massachusetts' general hospital. Johnson and Johnson not only fund much of Biederman's work, they also manufacture risperdal, one of the drugs that is commonly used in the treatment of children diagnosed with bipolar disorder. It is commonplace (although deeply problematic) for work that is in the interests of a pharmaceutical company to be funded by that company, but Biederman's links with industry go beyond those that have become accepted. Articles in the *New York Times* in 2008 and 2009 report on evidence unearthed during a congressional investigation that show that Biederman promised Johnson and Johnson that clinical trials he had yet to perform would show good results for their drug, and that he also failed to disclose to his university the full extent of his payments (Harris, 2008–2009). Big money is involved; between 2000 and 2007 Biederman received $1.6 million from drug companies. Biederman matters because he is one of the key researchers arguing that irritability in children may be regarded as equivalent to mania in adults. His work is cited in documents that discuss the deliberations of the committees revising the DSM.[2]

A paediatric variant of bipolar disorder was suggested for inclusion in the DSM-5 (Ghaemi et al., 2008), but instead the committees decided to include a new diagnosis, disruptive mood dysregulation disorder. The diagnostic criteria require that a child aged between six and eighteen at first diagnosis experiences temper outbursts three or more times per week, and has irritable mood between outbursts. Problematic symptoms must go on for at least twelve months, and must not be limited to a single setting (thus a child who only had outbursts at school would not receive a diagnosis). The aim of the new category is to provide a better label for many of those children who are currently being diagnosed with bipolar disorder (APA, 2013, p. 810). An explicit hope of the workgroup is that the new category will encourage research into different treatments, such that in time children receiving this diagnosis may receive therapy that is more appropriate than antipsychotics. Only time can tell whether the aim of limiting the treatment of children with antipsychotics will be achieved. The worry is that in being an apparently less severe diagnosis than bipolar disorder the new label will not simply be applied to those children who might previously have been diagnosed with bipolar disorder, but also more widely. If this occurs then the new category will only serve to increase the diagnosis of children and expand the market for pharmaceuticals (Axelson et al., 2011).

Note also that although there is no code for a paediatric variant of bipolar disorder, the DSM-5 still permits clinicians to make such diagnoses. The DSM-5 text advises that:

> The recognition that many individuals, particularly children and, to a lesser extent, adolescents, experience bipolar-like phenomena that do not meet the criteria for bipolar I, bipolar II, or cyclothymic disorder is reflected in the availability of the other specified bipolar and related disorder category. (APA, 2013, p. 123)

In contrast, the DSM-IV made no mention of bipolar disorders in children. The new suggestion, that a paediatric variant of bipolar disorder might be coded under bipolar disorder otherwise specified, goes a long way to legitimise the diagnosis. As we have seen in Chapter Two, some disorders that eventually come to be fully recognised, with their own diagnostic criteria, first make it into the DSM via being mentioned in the text.

With the splitting of depression into various subtypes, the introduction of disruptive mood dysregulation disorder, and the DSM's new claim that bipolar disorders in children might take atypical forms, we have cases where the DSM comes to be shaped by, and in reaction to, the interests of the drugs companies but via mechanisms that do not depend on the APA or DSM committee members directly receiving cash. In so far as research in psychiatry depends on industry money, over time viewpoints useful to industry are emphasised while those that are less useful become buried. As a consequence the "consensus view" that one arrives at by reviewing the psychiatric literature shifts in accord with the interests of industry. The influence of pharmaceutical funding on psychiatric research runs so deep that action by the APA will be inadequate to protect the DSM from its impact. Ultimately the only remedy that will safeguard against industry interests shaping the DSM will be for the evidence base to be created independently of industry influence—and this would require nothing less than a revolution in the way in which mental health research is funded.

Notes

1. A comparison of the websites of the National Alliance on Mental Illness (NAMI), the main US patient support group for mental disorder, with that of Mind, the main UK mental health charity, is suggestive. NAMI receives much funding from drug companies, and on its website tends to promote medication, while Mind does not accept donations from drugs companies. There have been allegations that NAMI has become overly influenced by industry donations, and in particular that Pfizer's donations to NAMI account for

the NAMI website mentioning that the antipsychotic drug Geodon might be used to treat children, even though the drug has not been approved by the Food and Drug Administration (FDA) in this age group (Edwards, 2009).

2. Referencing these documents is problematic. They were available on APA websites while the DSM-5 was under preparation, but along with all the draft criteria were removed prior to the DSM-5 being published.

CHAPTER THREE

Controversies of process: transparency and patient involvement

While the DSM is produced by the APA, transparency is bound to be problematic. The DSM is at one and the same time a document produced by a private organisation, and also one that has an impact on mental health practice worldwide. This creates a tension: the DSM is controlled by a smallish group of North American psychiatrists, but many would like to have an input into its creation.

In managing the systems via which the DSM is produced, the APA seeks to achieve a variety of mutually incompatible aims. The APA must make money from the DSM, protect the status of psychiatry relative to other mental health professions, maintain scientific respectability, ensure the cooperation of other mental health professionals in using the DSM, and maintain compatibility with the ICD (the classification published by the WHO). Some of these aims are best met by a revisionary process that is secret and dominated by the APA; others are best achieved by openness. Concerns about money and professional status encourage secrecy. Sales of the classification are essential to APA finances, and so it cannot afford for pirated copies of the manual to become too easily available.

Similarly the professional dominance of psychiatry can best be reaffirmed by making sure that psychiatrists are seen to be in the driving seat when it comes to constructing the classification. On the other hand, the manual will only be useful if it is widely adopted and is perceived to have credibility in the eyes of non-psychiatrists. This requires some level of cooperation from other mental health professionals and patient groups, which is best achieved via involvement and openness. Adding to the complexity, the APA cannot be understood as a purely self-interested organisation. The APA is complex, dynamic and internally conflicted. Some within the APA will always seek to "do the right thing", and will support moves they believe to be in the interests of patients even if these go against the narrow interests of organised psychiatry.

As I will show, the APA's strategies with regard to transparency and inclusion in the processes of DSM production, particularly with regard to patients, can only be understood when it is recognised that it is responding to conflicting goals.

The APA has found it comparatively easy to include other mental health professionals, and professionals from other countries, in the committees responsible for revising the DSM. About a third of workgroup members are non-psychiatrists (mainly psychologists) and thirty per cent are not US-based (Oldham, 2011).[1]

Incorporating patient views into the processes of DSM revision has proved much more controversial and problematic. The history of relations between the APA and patient groups has sometimes been strained. Most famously, during the late 1960s and early 1970s gay activists protested outside APA meetings in their quest to have homosexuality removed from the DSM (Bayer, 1981). On a lesser scale, protests by patients continue. In 2012 protesters employing the slogan "labels are for jars not people", protested against the DSM outside the APA annual meeting (Davies, 2012). The response to the protest nicely illustrates the internal diversity within the APA, and also some of the problems that face those who seek to establish meaningful dialogue between patients and professionals. After the protest, some of the protesters joined with psychiatrists at the radical caucus—an offshoot APA meeting. Reportedly, the "radical" psychiatrists were not radical enough for the protesters.

> David Oaks, from Mindfreedom, led the way by refusing to sit quietly while the Radical Caucus proceeded with business as usual. He stood up, he got angry, he yelled, he sang a song, he put on his red nose, and he pounded on the table. (Lewis, 2012)

In this description we catch a glimpse of some of the problems that are faced by those seeking dialogue. On the one hand we have psychiatrists: privileged, well educated, in this case well meaning, but professionally implicated in problematic histories. On the other hand, we have patient activists: in this instance, angry, and suspicious that polite academic discussion will achieve nothing. The barriers to debate are formidable.

The official line of the chairmen of the DSM-5 is that patient involvement in the development process is a good thing:

> We endorse the perspective that patients can and should play a more active role in the formation of diagnostic criteria for mental illnesses. (Regier, Kuhl, Kupfer, & McNulty, 2010, p. 308)

How were patients involved in the processes of DSM revision? A patient representative, James McNulty, past president of the NAMI, sat on the DSM-5 task force—but as a single patient representative amongst hundreds of committee members his presence is plausibly best understood as totemic.

More importantly, along with all other interested parties, patients were able to comment on drafts of the DSM published on the website.[2] The APA has promoted this as the primary means by which patients might have an input. The web-based consultation received a huge response. The APA received more than 13,000 comments, many from patients and their families, which were "systematically reviewed" by the relevant DSM work groups (APA, 2013, p. 8).

The APA website does not allow for the viewing of comments. A flavour can be gained from Suzy Chapman's website where she has sought to gather together comments about somatic symptom disorder (which is a category of great concern to many of those with chronic fatigue syndrome (CFS)/ME) (Chapman, 2012). The posts on her website vary from paper-length submissions from patient groups, to brief comments noting personal experiences from individual patients. Most comments seem well intentioned and well informed, but the overall feeling on reading them is one of repetition. Over and over again, those commenting on the proposed category express their concerns that it will lead to what they consider a physical illness being diagnosed as a psychiatric illness. The concerns of patients with CFS/ME are understandable, but it is hard to imagine what new information the DSM-5 workgroups might have gained from reading these comments: everyone involved already knew that this was a major concern for patients.

Perhaps the public consultation regarding drafts of the DSM-5 is best not thought of as an information gathering exercise. Efforts to include others in the revisionary process might be thought of as potentially seeking to achieve any of three, not necessarily incompatible, aims. First, consultation might aim at gaining information which might otherwise be overlooked by the DSM workgroups, and which might help improve the DSM. Second, consultation might aim at promoting a feeling of inclusion in those groups consulted. In so far as they have some "ownership" of the DSM, outsider groups might become more cooperative in using it. Third, consultation might be used to manage and dissolve dissent.

How processes of consultation might be used to manage dissent perhaps requires some explanation. In outline, the process would be as follows. It is predictable that many will get upset about proposed changes to the DSM. In the past, their only option was to seek to influence the APA by unruly means. The provision of an official approved mechanism for expressing dissent renders such protests less likely. Those who are unhappy with the DSM can view drafts, and file a comment. Once a comment has been filed they are told that the APA is very grateful for their input, that the committees will carefully review their suggestions, and are reminded that the draft is just a working document and may well be revised. While it is left unclear exactly what happens to comments, in so far as dissenters have been given the opportunity to participate in the revisionary process, they have nothing to protest about. They go away, hopefully quietly, to wait and see what happens.

Processes for consultation often aim at achieving all three of these aims—information gathering, promoting inclusion, and managing dissent—at the same time. However, depending on the aim that dominates, the precise mechanisms for consultation may be expected to differ. If a consultation genuinely aims to gather information, then it makes sense to try to ensure that the comments of those consulted are as well informed as possible. How might this be achieved? Most obviously, as much relevant information as possible will be shared with those consulted. One would also expect that those consulted would be supported in educating themselves, and in refining their deliberations: all of us think better if we have the opportunity to test out our ideas in discussion with others. On the other hand, if the aims of consultation are primarily to foster feelings of inclusion, or to manage dissent, it will not be so important for the comments of those consulted to be well informed. At the extreme, if no one is really interested in gaining information from comments, then it doesn't matter what they say: comments are received, commentators are thanked, comments are filed away, job done.

The online facility for commenting on drafts of the DSM-5 only partially accorded with what one would hope for if the primary aim of the consultation were to gather information. It is true that in revising the DSM-5 the APA made an unprecedented amount of information freely available to members of the public. However, not all the information in the APA's possession that might have been useful to commentators was made available. In particular the data gathered in field trials regarding the reliability and prevalence of new categories was only published once the period for consultation was over. This data was a matter of key concern for many patient communities. Perhaps more significantly, those posting comments were unable to view the comments made by others, and as such they were unable to develop their comments in the light of what had already been said.

Considering its actions more widely, the APA has not been entirely supportive of attempts to develop informed patient-led discussion of the DSM. The case of Suzy Chapman stands out. Chapman became one of the most read bloggers monitoring the DSM revision process. She is a UK-based patient advocate, associated with the ME/chronic fatigue syndrome community. Her blog started with the name *DSM5watch.wordpress.com* and gathered a broad following. In December 2011 Chapman was threatened with legal action by the APA who claimed she was violating their trademark rights by using the name DSM-5 (Chapman, no date). The APA action met with widespread condemnation, and was generally seen as an attempt by the APA to censor debate about the DSM-5 (e.g., Frances, 2012a; Heisel, 2012). As another example, Paula Caplan describes her experience of a conference call for patient advocates with DSM-5 officials in which she participated (Caplan, 2011). Her efforts to coordinate the questions of the activists prior to the call were hindered: the APA refused to forward an email from her to other participants, or to share their contact details. The call was dominated by speakers for the APA, and many patient advocates did not get a chance to speak. Such actions seem to aim to close down, rather than promote, informed, patient-led discussion, and are hard to understand if the APA wholeheartedly wanted patients to be able to play a meaningful role in discussions surrounding the DSM-5.

The mechanisms employed by the APA in managing the debates about the DSM suggest that it is not yet fully committed to involving patients in revising the DSM. Still, greater patient involvement in future editions of the DSM can be expected. Many within the APA genuinely desire greater patient involvement, and external political pressure for patient involvement is likely to increase. Patients also have the potential to make a useful contribution to future editions of the manual. While I believe that patients have a useful contribution to make to the DSM, I suggest that soliciting comments from individual patients (as was done with the online comment facility) cannot be the best way to enable this contribution. The DSM affects millions of people worldwide: in this context finding out that Jim Johnson from Dallas would rather be spoken of as having Asperger's disorder rather than autism spectrum disorder should be neither here nor there. Patients have an important role to play but this must either be considered en masse as stakeholders (e.g., as one of the 10,000 patients who prefer "Asperger's" as a label), or as patient-researchers.

The idea that patient-researchers might contribute to future editions of the DSM needs some defence. Robert Spitzer, chairman of the DSM-III, considers such suggestions "politically correct nonsense" (Spitzer, 2004). What exactly is it that I think patient-researchers might offer?

First, let's clarify what I mean by "patient-researcher". I mean a researcher, who uses the normal methods of research, but who also happens to be, or to have been, a patient. Such people have much to contribute not only to DSM revision, but to mental health research in general. Over recent decades research in science studies has confirmed what common sense already knew: it matters who does research (see, for example, Cooper, 2007, ch. 8; Haraway, 1989; Longino, 1990). How science is done—who gets a say, what issues are investigated, what results are valued—is always a political issue; those with different interests answer such questions differently. The end result is that those who work for industry will tend to find results that promote the interests of industry, while patient-researchers will be more likely to find results that promote the interests of patients.

Let's turn away from the DSM for a moment, to consider an example of the sort of beneficial influence patient-researchers can have on research in mental health. In the UK a "yellow card" system whereby health professionals can alert the Committee of Safety in Medicine to suspected adverse drug reactions has long been in use. Patients taking psychoactive medications were concerned that their experiences of drug reactions, which they reported to clinicians, were not always being passed on to the committee. In response, Mind, the UK mental health charity, collected reports of drug reactions from patients and published summaries in 1996 and 2001 (Cobb, 1996; Cobb, Darton, & Juttla, 2001). These reports helped highlight concerns about SSRI use potentially being linked to feelings of violence and suicide. Since the Mind reports, these concerns have been taken up by mainstream researchers, and the procedure for reporting adverse drug reactions in the UK has changed so that patients can now directly report suspected reactions. Here we can see clearly that the interests and assumptions of researchers led them to do research differently. In a case where some patients had reported troubling feelings following drug use, mainstream medics tended to dismiss the patient reports. Industry-researchers actually had data that suggested that SSRIs plausibly induced suicidal thought in some patients, but, as from their point of view this was an unwanted result, they massaged their published findings to disguise this link (Healy, 2006). Mind took the suspicions seriously, trusted patients to report their own experiences, and thought links between SSRI use and suicidal thoughts worth publishing.

Turning to consider the DSM directly, greater patient-researcher involvement could be expected to have similarly beneficial effects. Patient-researchers have a valuable role to play in revising the DSM because their background and interests will make it more likely that they will spot mistakes that can be missed by committees made up of clinicians and researchers. Let's consider some concrete examples. In Chapter One I described a change in the wording of the diagnostic criteria for phobias that I suggested must be a mistake. Previously patients had to recognise their fears as unreasonable, now the clinician has to judge the patient's fear to be out of proportion. I suggested that this would make it possible for someone with rational fears to be diagnosed merely because their fears were based on information about which the clinician was ignorant. How could such an implication be missed? Plausibly the error here arose because the committee overlook the possibility that a patient might know more than a clinician. This is the sort of error that patient-researchers would be less likely to make. To point forward to another example, in the next chapter, we will see that when revisions are made to the DSM the committees are supposed to consider social and political consequences; only revisions that on balance do no harm are to be accepted. In considering whether this criterion is met, when a new disorder is proposed, committees consider factors such as the likelihood that the disorder will be misused, and that patients will be stigmatised. As we'll see, when it comes to hoarding disorder, I think the committee got this calculation wrong. I'd expect patient-researchers to be more sensitive to the malign effects of diagnosis than are clinicians.

At present, there are not enough patient-researchers, but their numbers are growing. It's reasonable to hope that by the time the DSM next comes to be revised a critical mass of patient-researchers will have become established, such that patient-researchers might play a significant role in the processes of DSM revision by sitting alongside other experts on the committees responsible for revisions.

Notes

1. Less effectively, the routine clinical practice field trials (where draft criteria were tested in small practices) were also supposed to offer professionals from other mental health professions a chance to contribute to discussions around the construction of the DSM (Brauser, 2011; Kupfer, 2012). However, although the trials were originally designed to involve nearly 5,000 clinicians from a variety of backgrounds (APA, 2011), only 621 clinicians actually participated. (Mościcki, 2013).
2. The APA has now removed the drafts.

CHAPTER FOUR

Issues of content: the birth of a new diagnosis—hoarding disorder

This chapter focuses on one of the new additions to the DSM-5 that has garnered the least discussion. It will act as an illustration of how changes to the DSM come about, what impact they may have, and how even the least controversial of them can be problematic.

Hoarding disorder is included as a separate disorder for the first time in the DSM-5. In the DSM-IV, hoarding is mentioned only as a possible symptom of obsessive-personality disorder. The campaign to have hoarding upgraded to a recognised distinct disorder started some time ago. In 1996, a key researcher in the area, Randy Frost, together with Tamara Hartl, published a paper on hoarding that included criteria for the disorder's diagnosis. They suggested that clinical compulsive hoarding might be defined on the basis of

> (1) the acquisition of, and failure to discard, a large number of possessions that appear to be useless or of limited value; (2) living spaces sufficiently cluttered so as to preclude activities for which those spaces were designed; and (3) significant distress or impairment in functioning caused by the hoarding. (Frost & Hartl, 1996, p. 341)

Notably this definition meets the style of diagnostic criteria included in the DSM-IV. The criteria "operationalise" the condition: that is, they state as clearly as possible what sorts of observable behaviour must occur for the condition to be diagnosed. The "distress or impairment" condition is also characteristic of the DSM-IV diagnostic criteria sets: most of the sets of diagnostic criteria require distress or impairment before a condition can be diagnosed. The criteria proposed by Frost and Hartl were taken up by other researchers, and over the last two decades interest in the disorder has grown rapidly.

At the same time, interest in the condition developed amongst patient groups. One of the key patient support groups for those with OCD is the International OCD Foundation. The International OCD Foundation is well organised. Its website is large, attractively designed, and informative (http://www.ocfoundation.org/). In 2010 the International OCD Foundation launched a section of its website, called Hoarding Center. The Hoarding Center discusses a range of different possible treatments for hoarding, including a structured cognitive-behavioural approach developed by Frost (the researcher who first published proposed diagnostic criteria). Further interest in the disorder has been fostered by the media. Highly visual, hoarding provokes both fascination and revulsion and has become a staple of reality TV. In the US, the A&E series *Hoarders* started in 2009, and is now in its sixth season. Slightly behind, by 2012, the UK had multiple hoarding series: Channel 4 aired *Obsessive Compulsive Hoarder* and *The Hoarder Next Door*. BBC1 offered *Britain's Biggest Hoarder*.

The result of all this activity was that by the time the DSM-5 was being drafted the idea that hoarding was a serious, prevalent, and distinct mental disorder had already become widespread. As discussed in the Introduction and later in Chapter Two, one should always be alert to possible links between the interests of the pharmaceutical industry and changes to the DSM. In the case of hoarding, researchers and patient groups involved in raising awareness of the condition appear to have no links with the pharmaceutical industry. This being said, now hoarding disorder has appeared in the DSM, the pharmaceutical industry has lost no time in starting drug trials (Wieczner, 2013). Hoarding disorder has an estimated prevalence of up to six per cent, providing a huge market for any company that manages to get a drug approved for its treatment (APA, 2013, p. 249).

The diagnostic criteria for hoarding disorder included in the DSM-5 are very similar to those first suggested by Frost and Hartl in their 1996 paper. Whenever a new disorder is included in the DSM, a rationale for its inclusion is provided. In the case of hoarding, the relevant literature review was published in *Depression and Anxiety* (Mataix-Cols et al., 2010). In making a case for the diagnosis to be included in the DSM three hurdles had to be cleared—scientific, conceptual, and ethical. First, the key scientific question: is hoarding a distinct condition, or should it be thought of only as a possible symptom of other disorders? Second, the conceptual issue: does hoarding satisfy the definition of mental disorder included in the DSM? Third, an ethical question: is the inclusion of hoarding in the DSM likely to do more good than harm? Let's consider each of these requirements in greater detail.

First, the scientific hurdle: the review asked whether hoarding could be considered a valid disorder. In particular, it weighed the evidence that hoarding can properly be considered a distinct condition from obsessive-compulsive disorder (OCD). A number of studies suggested key differences between hoarding and OCD. The two conditions are experienced differently by patients: while obsessive thoughts are typically experienced as intrusive, thoughts associated with hoarding normally fit coherently with a patient's other thoughts and values. There seem to be differences in natural history: while hoarding typically gets worse over a patient's lifetime, OCD does not. Neuroimaging studies suggest distinctions between hoarders and those with OCD. Treatment response may differ in that people with OCD tend to be more responsive to treatment with SSRIs, and exposure and ritual prevention. Taken together, there seems fair evidence that hoarding and OCD are distinct.

The paper then tackles the second hurdle: does hoarding fit the DSM definition of disorder? The DSM definition was first included in the DSM-III and remained substantially unchanged through to DSM-IV-TR. As set out in DSM-IV-TR, the definition requires that

> ... each of the mental disorders is conceptualised as a clinically significant behavioral or psychological syndrome or pattern that occurs in an individual and that is associated with present distress (e.g., a painful symptom) or disability (i.e., impairment in one or more important areas of functioning) or with significantly increased risk of suffering death, pain, disability, or an important loss of freedom ... Whatever its original cause, it must currently be considered a manifestation of a behavioral, psychological, or biological dysfunction in the individual. Neither deviant behavior (e.g., political, religious, or sexual) nor conflicts that are primarily between the individual and society are mental disorders unless the deviance or conflict is a symptom of a dysfunction in the individual, as described above. (APA, 2000, p. xxxi)

The review paper goes through the DSM definition point by point to see if hoarding can be made to fit: that is, it considers whether there is a syndrome, whether it causes distress or impairment, and whether the condition might better be thought of as a clash between individual values and the social context. The issues of distress or impairment, and of clashes of values, are especially problematic. Many hoarders deny that they have a problem: they may not see their hoard as junk, but as stuff that they will one day use. Faced with such difficulties, the review authors decide to interpret "distress or impairment" liberally. They conclude that the criterion is often met as hoarding can pose a health hazard, and lead to conflicts with others. They note, for example, that "8–12% of hoarding participants had been evicted or threatened with eviction at some point in their lives" (Mataix-Cols et al., 2010, p. 565). The reviewers see the conflict between hoarder and society as being rooted in a problem in the hoarder: "Given the evidence of associated impairment and underlying disturbance, it seems clear that compulsive hoarding is not solely a result of social deviance or conflicts with society." (Mataix-Cols et al., 2010, p. 566).

The final hurdle that hoarding had to clear before being included in the DSM was ethical. Guidelines for those revising the DSM demand that proposers should consider whether "the harm that arises from the adoption of the proposed diagnosis exceed[s] the benefit that would accrue to affected individuals" (Kendler, Kupfer, Narrow, Phillips, & Fawcett, 2009). Only revisions that on balance do no harm are to be accepted. The reviewers briefly discuss the potential harms and benefits of including hoarding disorder in the DSM. They conclude that on balance the new diagnosis can be hoped helpful in that it will "likely increase public awareness, improve identification of cases, and stimulate both research and the development of specific treatments for hoarding disorder" (Mataix-Cols et al., 2010, p. 556).

The review paper ends by concluding that hoarding should be included in the DSM-5, and suggests that the prevalence of the new condition might be two to five per cent. The addition of hoarding disorder in the DSM-5 will make a difference around the world. With news that the condition would be included in the DSM, state authorities in Australia started developing policies on how to respond to hoarding problems in the community (no author, 2012), and patient groups in the UK predicted that help from the NHS would become easier to access (Mataix-Cols, no date).

I have a number of interconnected concerns about the inclusion of hoarding disorder. First let's remember that patterns of consumption and waste disposal have varied radically across place and time, and differ between individuals. Susan Strasser's (1999) *Waste and Want: A Social History of Trash* makes it clear that there is nothing that is unambiguously rubbish. Whether one sees stuff as raw material or useless depends on what one can imagine doing with it, and powers of imagination vary radically with class, age, gender, and occupation. Most obviously, poor people have always seen value in what the rich throw away. Strasser points out that those who can make items tend also to see how to mend them—thus ripped clothes look like rags only to those with no dressmaking skills. Whether something has value varies also with changing industrial processes: where paper is made from rags, and fertiliser from bones, rags and bones have monetary value. As a result of such variation, those who have lived under different norms, either because they are older, or have moved geographically, can easily find their own patterns of consumption and waste to be out of sync with those who live around them. The variation in practices means that whether someone is "hoarding junk" is not a straightforwardly factual matter because "what is rubbish to some is useful or valuable to others" (Strasser, 1999, p. 9).

Strasser's work also makes it clear that DSM-style hoarding can occur only within a very particular cultural niche. We live in cultures of plenty and consumption, where it is common for much to be thrown away. Many, living in other parts of the world, do not. Even in Europe and the US, for most people, it only became possible to hoard junk around the mid-nineteenth century. Prior to then, people had little and wasted less. Whole industries were devoted to re-using the sorts of "worthless trash" that hoarders are now condemned for keeping. There were traders in bones, in used bottles, rags, and paper. Getting large quantities of such objects would be difficult, and if achieved such collections would not have been considered worthless. Not only materially, but also conceptually, "junk" did not yet exist; the word "junk", used in the sense of "worthless objects", first appeared only in 1841.

Still, although rubbish may be relative, and although hoarding has not always been possible, shouldn't we admit that those who fill their houses from floor to ceiling with precarious piles of newspapers and boxes have a mental health problem? I accept that the relationship between hoarder and possessions is unusual, and also think that it is unwise to fill one's house with junk, but I am still not entirely convinced that hoarding is best thought of as a mental health problem. Remember, first, that there are many habits and behaviours that are unwise but that we do not pathologise. For example, many of us reduce our life expectancy by years because we fail to exercise or to eat healthily. Others fail to back up computer files, or to save adequately for old age. Maybe hoarding differs from such examples of folly in that hoarding is more unusual, but rarity in itself cannot transform a pattern of behaviour from a bad habit into a disorder.

Those who consider hoarding a disorder will likely point out that it is associated with distinctive patterns of brain activity, and can be further distinguished from "normal behaviour" by its natural history, treatment response, and the way in which it seems to run in families. But we should note that none of these natural facts can clearly distinguish a disorder from a normal (though in this case unwise) pattern of behaviour. Normal behaviours, for example playing music, may also be accompanied by distinctive patterns of brain activity (Schlaug, 2003), can be affected by psychoactive drugs (Fachner, 2006), have a distinctive natural history (Gembris, 2006), and run in families (Pulli et al., 2008).

Whether hoarding should be considered a disorder must depend also on whether we consider it to be the sort of problem that is appropriately dealt with by medical means, and here we should pause. Medical treatment implicitly takes the root cause of a problem to be located "within" an individual,[1] but problematic hoarding clearly arises only in certain environments. Consider the finding that one of the key factors that distinguishes those who meet the diagnostic criteria for hoarding disorder from sub-threshold cases is that those who are sub-threshold "were more likely to live in larger properties that had, on average, an additional room" (Mataix-Cols, Billotti, Fernández de la Cruz, & Nordsletten, 2013, p. 842). Here we see that hoarding problems arise relationally—the combination of individual characteristics, living situation, and broader material and social environment, results in problems. It is plausibly the case that if hoarders were psychologically different they wouldn't hoard. But equally, if they had bigger houses, or a rag and bone man periodically came round and offered them money to take away their collected waste, there wouldn't be a hoarding problem either.

We should also worry about the fact that hoarders are said to often "lack insight"—that is they don't think they have a problem, and they don't want to be helped. Remember that new disorders are supposed to be added to the DSM only if they are likely to do more good than harm. The addition of hoarding disorder to the DSM will facilitate the diagnosis and treatment of those who do not want to be diagnosed or treated. It is worth reminding ourselves that treating those who "lack insight" is generally a nasty business, and frequently involves tears and arguments. I am not suggesting that all hoarders should be left alone. Certainly it is true that sometimes an individual's possessions will need reining in by others. A vermin-ridden, or structurally unsound, house must be dealt with; children cannot be left to live in faeces-filled dwellings. But there are already laws for dealing with such problems. My worry is that in medicalising hoarding, the threshold for coercive intervention will become much lower. The risk is that rather than intervention being thought justified only when the welfare of others is at risk, "help" will be provided in much less severe cases for the hoarder's "own good".

It is easy to criticise, harder to make positive suggestions. If I think including hoarding disorder as a new category in the DSM was a mistake, what would I have recommended instead? At present, forms of cognitive-behavioural therapy are amongst the most promising treatments being developed for hoarding. For example, with colleagues, Randy Frost has developed a self-help support group programme called the Buried in Treasures workshop (Frost, Ruby, & Shuer, 2012). Hoarders meet with other hoarders, discuss a chapter from the accompanying book, and complete weekly exercises dealing with acquisition, discarding, and disorganisation. Initial trials suggest the therapy is highly effective. If Frost's programme works, then this is great news. But there is no need to think of this as "therapy", it could equally be framed as a structured and peer-supported programme for dealing with a bad habit (rather like Weight Watchers). Hoarding often doesn't need to be pathologised before hoarders can be helped.

This being said, I accept that there may be some hoarders who do require medical help (possibly because their hoarding is associated with some other mental disorder). However, any individual hoarders for whom medical help would be useful could have been diagnosed, using the "other" codes, without it having been added to the DSM as a distinct disorder.

Finally, I should emphasise that although I think hoarding might often be better considered a bad habit than a disorder, I do not think that this also applies across the board to other diagnoses added to the DSM. Each condition added to the DSM is unique, and I would wish to distance myself from any generalised "anti-psychiatry" critique of the DSM.

Note

1. It is true that many family therapists use relational diagnoses, but the status of "disorders" that are not conceived of as being located within an individual remains problematic.

CHAPTER FIVE

Issues of content: the changing limits of autistic spectrum disorders

This chapter tells a story of changes in definitions, of prevalence rates, and of costs, all entwined. The headline news with regard to autism and related conditions is that Asperger's disorder has been removed as a standalone diagnosis from the DSM-5. Instead the new category autistic spectrum disorder (ASD) includes most of those previously diagnosed with autism as well as most of those previously diagnosed with Asperger's disorder. Also subsumed into ASD are the DSM-IV diagnoses of Rett's disorder—a rare genetic condition; and PDD-NOS—pervasive developmental disorder not otherwise specified—a ragbag code for those with autism-like disorders who didn't fulfil the criteria for any specific disorder.

Amongst researchers, whether Asperger's should be considered to be a distinct condition, or merely the mildest form of autism, continues to be a source of contention (for a review see Matson & Wilkins, 2008). With the changes to the DSM-5, at least for the time being, those who advocate that there is no distinction between Asperger's and high-functioning autism have won. The committees responsible for the change argue that the distinctions between Asperger's, autism, and PDD-NOS imposed by the DSM-IV could not be reliably drawn. DSM-IV criteria for Asperger's require that early language development is normal, but as most children are only diagnosed in later childhood or adolescence, it can be hard for parents to remember whether this was the case (Happé, 2011). One study found that many children diagnosed with Asperger's disorder did not actually meet DSM-IV criteria (Williams et al., 2008), and another that whether a child would be diagnosed with Asperger's disorder or autism depended to a large extent on which clinic they visited (Lord et al., 2012). The aim now is to stop trying to "carve meatloaf at the joints" (Happé, 2011, p. 541). What may well turn out to be more important than the lumping together of diagnoses, however, is that the revisions to the DSM may affect the overall rates of those diagnosed with some sort of autism-related disorder.

The effect that the changes to the DSM will have on overall prevalence rates (i.e., the DSM-IV autism-like disorders lumped together versus new ASD) is hard to predict. Traditionally, and in the DSM-IV, the key difference between children with autism and with Asperger's was that those with Asperger's showed no significant delays in early language skills, while those with autism developed language late, if at all. In merging the disorders, in DSM-5, the criteria relating to problems with language development, previously included in the DSM-IV as symptoms of autism, have been removed. Other changes in diagnostic criteria have also been made, for example, in the age by which symptoms must be manifest. The multiple differences between DSM-IV and DSM-5 make it hard to tell whether a larger or smaller group of people can be expected to meet the new criteria.

Preliminary studies seeking to find out how many of the patients who met DSM-IV criteria will also meet DSM-5 criteria have reported inconsistent results. Based on analyses using draft DSM-5 criteria, some studies predicted that a significant number of those diagnosed under DSM-IV would no longer be diagnosed (Dickerson Mayes, Black, & Tierney, 2013; Matson, Belva, Horovitz, Kozlowski, & Bamburg, 2012; Mattila et al.,

2011). On the other hand, a study frequently cited by members of the DSM committees found "most children with DSM-IV diagnoses will meet DSM-5 criteria" (Huerta, Bishop, Duncan, Hus, & Lord, 2012, p. 1056). All these studies were limited in their design. A key problem is that they sought to estimate the numbers that would satisfy DSM-5 criteria but depended on rating scales developed to operationalise DSM-IV criteria. As such, some symptoms given greater prominence in the DSM-5 were not adequately probed.

One of the aims of the DSM field trial was to estimate the effect that revisions will have on prevalence rates. In the field trials, data from two different hospitals was used to estimate the prevalence of autism-related disorders under the DSM-IV and the DSM-5. The trials found some decrease at one site, which was partly accounted for by some of those who would have had DSM-IV autism-related diagnoses receiving a diagnosis of social (or pragmatic) communication disorder under the DSM-5 (Regier et al., 2013, p. 67). Social communication disorder is a diagnosis new to the DSM-5 for individuals whose problems stem chiefly from difficulties in pragmatics. Crucially it is grouped with other communication disorders (stuttering etc.) rather than with autism. This matters, as we shall see later, because when it comes to the provision of services not all mental health diagnoses are equal.

The field trial design had its weaknesses. Notably the total number of children with ASD studied in the field trial was rather small—thirty-seven at one site, thirty-one at the other (Clarke et al., 2013, p. 51). More importantly there is reason to think that the results of field trials, no matter how good their design, can turn out to be a poor predictor of changes in prevalence rates that will occur later on. Field trials were run prior to the publication of the DSM-IV (Volkmar et al., 1994). These predicted that the introduction of Asperger's and changes to the autism criteria would make little difference to prevalence rates. In reality, since the DSM-IV there has been a massive increase in autism-related diagnoses. For example, in Utah, prevalence increased 100% from 2002–2008, such that by 2008 one in every seventy-seven children aged eight was being diagnosed with ASD (Pinborough-Zimmerman et al., 2012). This increase is due to a range of factors—a broadening of diagnostic criteria, changes in the likelihood of detection, an earlier average age of diagnosis, and also, possibly, a genuine increase in the underlying causes of autism (Leonard et al., 2010).

As awareness of autism and Asperger's has increased, parents have become more likely to seek these diagnoses, and clinicians have become more likely to make them. It is important to bear in mind that work has to be done by patients (or in this case their parents) before diagnoses are made (Liu, King, & Bearman, 2010). At a minimum, parents have to bring their children to a clinician in order to achieve a diagnosis. Often, at first presentation, they will be frustrated in one way or another—a child will be referred to others, parents may be told that nothing is wrong, and so on. Siklos and Kerns (2007) found that children who eventually received an autism-related diagnosis were first seen by an average of 4.5 professionals, a process that typically took three years.

When a child is diagnosed, there is often some leeway in the diagnosis that is given. At the "lower-functioning" end, autistic spectrum disorders can be hard to distinguish from intellectual disability. At the "higher-functioning" extreme, they blend into normal oddity. Physicians tend to favour diagnoses that they judge helpful, and which diagnoses are helpful varies with context. Parents also have some input into the diagnoses that get made: for example, parents may seek out clinicians who are known to favour a particular diagnosis.

Whether a diagnosis of an autism-related disorder has been desirable has varied as the cultural stereotypes associated with these conditions, and the services that are provided for them, have changed. During the 1960s and 1970s, psychodynamic theories that blamed "refrigerator mothers" for autism meant that many parents were not keen on their child receiving an autism diagnosis (Liu, King, & Bearman, 2010). Since then, biological theories of causation have gained wide acceptance, and autism has become relatively destigmatised as a diagnosis. Until the 1990s, many insurance companies had exemptions for autism (Peele, Lave, & Kelleher, 2002) and it was noted that "providers subsequently may choose not to use ASD diagnostic codes" (Pinborough-Zimmerman et al., 2012, p. 528). Times have changed, and these days, in many locations, services for children with autism are now better than those for children with intellectual disabilities. A friendly clinician faced with a borderline case will now likely write autism on the necessary forms.

Rates of diagnosis shift with awareness of a condition, the beliefs that surround it, and local levels of services. This means that predictions about the numbers that will come to be diagnosed once an edition of the DSM has been in use for some years are always uncertain. Still, prevalence rates matter hugely, particularly in the case of conditions such as autism-related disorders where costly therapies are indicated. As legal systems and bureaucracies use DSM categories to determine eligibility for services, if a child ceases to fulfil revised diagnostic criteria, this doesn't just mean a simple amendment to their medical records. The loss of a diagnosis can mean that the child risks losing educational and therapeutic services. Treatment for children with autism-related diagnoses often involves hours and hours of one-to-one supportive therapy. The cost means that a constant battle is waged between parents and advocates seeking to gain coverage for treatment, and providers and bureaucrats seeking to limit it.[1]

Arguments about service provision interact with debates about diagnostic thresholds—when thresholds are lowered, more people are diagnosed, and more people thus become eligible for services. In a number of interviews, David Kupfer, chair of the DSM-5 task force, has said that the DSM-5 aimed to reduce the numbers diagnosed with ASD and thus to reduce costs. In a 2010 interview he noted that combining autism, Asperger's, and PDD-NOS is an "unpopular proposal" but concluded, "but we have to do something about the rising rates of several childhood psychiatric disorders and this is an important adjustment to decrease the level of children with autism" (Verhoeff, 2010). Similarly, in a 2012 interview with the *New York Times* Kupfer maintained the same line: "We have to make sure not everybody who is a little odd gets a diagnosis of autism or Asperger disorder … It involves a use of treatment resources. It becomes a cost issue." (Harmon, 2012).

We should pause before taking Kupfer's comments to accurately reflect the intended aim (and still less the actual result) of the DSM revisions. As task force chair, Kupfer is a powerful man, but he does not have absolute control over the DSM revision process, which relies on a complex committee structure. Some of those on the work group revising autism-related conditions denied that they intended to restrict services (Happé, 2011; Singer, 2012), and in a 2012 news release the APA claimed that "despite what some critics have suggested, the issue of containing autism rates was not considered by the Work Group, nor was it a factor in revising the criteria" (Martin, 2012).

Patient and family support groups for those affected by autism-related conditions are well informed and well organised, and have been alert to the potential ramifications of changes to DSM criteria on service provision. A report by the Autistic Self Advocacy Network considered possible consequences of the proposed changes to diagnostic criteria (Ne'eman & Kapp, 2012). The report notes that some of those who were diagnosed with Asperger's or PDD-NOS under the DSM-IV will meet criteria for a DSM-5 diagnosis of ASD. The report judges that life should be made easier for these individuals: many services are currently available only to those with autism, and not to those with Asperger's or PDD-NOS. With the DSM-5, such divisions will be impossible. On the other hand, some who had DSM-IV diagnoses of Asperger's or PDD-NOS will not meet criteria for a DSM-5 diagnosis of ASD. Under the DSM-5 some of these people might be diagnosed with social communication disorder, but as this condition would not be grouped with ASD, the report worries that services for those so diagnosed might well be reduced.

Advocacy groups for autism-related conditions are seldom united. There are frequently tensions between high-functioning individuals with Asperger's and parents of lower-functioning children with autism. These groups have few needs in common. For the most part, however, autism groups came together to voice concerns that some of those with DSM-IV autism-related diagnoses might not be diagnosed under DSM-5. Petitions argued that broad definitions of ASD should be maintained, and advocates organised for the APA to be bombarded with emails and phone calls protesting against the proposed changes (Greenberg, 2013, pp. 296–299).

In the end, the move to maintain coverage for those with DSM-IV diagnoses won out. The DSM-5 diagnostic criteria includes a note that states that "Individuals with a well-established DSM-IV diagnosis of autistic disorder, Asperger's disorder, or pervasive developmental disorder not otherwise specified should be given the diagnosis of autism spectrum disorder" (APA, 2013, p. 51). This note is extraordinary, and unprecedented in the DSM. Given that there are clear differences between the old diagnostic criteria and the new, the claim that historical diagnoses can be maintained is quite clearly a compromise that aims at retaining services for those diagnosed under the DSM-IV.

There is a further and yet more remarkable footnote: PDD-NOS was one of a handful of diagnoses where the criteria were revised between DSM-IV and DSM-IV-TR. In the DSM-IV as a result of "an editorial mistake" (an "or" instead of an "and") diagnosis was theoretically possible in the absence of problems with social interaction (First & Pincus, 2002). Thus, it was possible for an individual whose sole symptom was "stereotyped behaviour, interests, and activities" to be diagnosed. The description was tightened in DSM-IV-TR (APA, 2000, p. 830). It is questionable whether the DSM-IV mistake would have had much impact. Few clinicians read the DSM carefully enough to spot the difference between an "and" and an "or", and paradigmatic cases of PDD-NOS would be those with an autism-like condition that is sub-threshold, or of unusually late onset. Still, in principle, fossilising DSM-IV diagnoses of PDD-NOS fossilises not only diagnoses made on the basis of old criteria but those made on the basis of a copyediting error.

The case of ASD illustrates how lobbying by activist groups can affect the DSM. Here diagnostic criteria have been revised in part on the basis of demands by patient groups. We also see how DSM diagnoses get entwined with questions of service provision. Prevalence rates matter hugely for questions of health policy, and individuals' lives are radically affected by whether they receive, or lose, a DSM diagnosis. Decisions about revisions to the DSM have to be guided by estimates as to how prevalence rates will be affected—but as rates of diagnosis depend not only on the wording of diagnostic criteria but also on the social and economic contexts in which diagnoses come to be made, these estimates regarding likely prevalence are no more than guesses, and frequently turn out to be radically wrong. Plausibly increasing awareness that massive unforeseen problems can occur post-publication has led to the revisions of recent editions being rather conservative. Committee members now know that changes can produce unpredictable problems, and so changes are avoided as much as possible.

Note

1. Although battles over the provision of services commonly occur with most mental health diagnoses, due to the related costs, those that surround autism treatment are perhaps

particularly nasty, and on occasion take a Kafkaesque turn. Consider this report on the ways in which legally mandated Medicaid waiver programmes (that are supposed to provide therapy) can operate in practice.

> States are allowed to cap the number of people who can enrol in these programs. In some states, enrolment waiting lists for the waiver programs are several years long. Because some autism interventions have been found to be effective only when applied by a certain early age, children with autism who remain on waiting lists for several years may exceed the eligible age range for the intervention before they can enrol in the waiver program. Officials in one state told us the average length of time a person is on the waiting list for either its autism or developmental disability waiver program exceeds 5 years. This state requires that a specific intensive one-on-one intervention be covered under its autism waiver program; however, state officials told us that in practice no child has ever received the service through the Medicaid waiver program. Because a child must receive the intervention by age six, and children are not usually diagnosed with autism until age three, by the time they come off the waiting list, they are no longer eligible for the intervention. (Government Accountability Office, 2006, p. 25)

CHAPTER SIX

The field trials: DSM-5 and the new crisis of reliability

At time of writing, the DSM-5 has only just been published, and studies showing what differences the revisions have made to clinical practice, research, or service provision, are unavailable. The DSM-5 field trials are currently the best estimators of likely effects. This chapter focuses on one particular issue that has become controversial following the field trials: reliability.

The diagnosis that a patient receives should depend on the symptoms, rather than on who does the diagnosing. Suppose a patient sees a clinical social worker in the United States and is judged to have schizophrenia. If a reliable classification system is used then it should enable, say, a psychiatrist in Kenya, to decide on the same diagnosis.

When the DSM-III was published in 1980, it was presented as solving the problem of ensuring diagnostic reliability (APA, 1980, pp. 467–472). The story told was that while in the dark days of psychoanalytic dominance a patient judged neurotic by one therapist might well appear psychotic or normal to another, with the employment of the DSM-III patients could expect to be given the same diagnosis by all clinicians. Proof of improvement was taken to be shown by a statistical measure, Cohen's kappa, which assesses the chances that two clinicians will agree on a diagnostic label. As DSM-III, and its successors, demonstrated "acceptable" values of kappa, the reliability problem was widely deemed to have been solved.

But then with reliability tests in the field trials of DSM-5 diagnostic criteria, something odd happened. In reports of the DSM-5 field trials, results that found kappas at values which for thirty-five years would have been judged "poor" or "unacceptable" suddenly became "good". Commentators with long memories pointed out the inconsistency (1 Boring Old Man, 2012; Frances, 2012b; Spitzer, Williams, & Endicott, 2012).

What had happened? Is the reliability of the DSM-5 really no better than that of classifications fifty years ago? What is truly a good value for kappa? And how much does the reliability of psychiatric diagnosis matter anyway? Let's go back and look at the debates in more detail to answer these questions.

The reliability of psychiatric diagnosis started to be a matter of some concern in the 1960s and 1970s. A number of studies sought to investigate the issue of reliability. Comparing the results of the different studies was difficult, as different studies employed different statistics and it was unclear what level of agreement one might reasonably expect (for a review of the debates see Kirk & Kutchins, 1992). Those who produced these early studies were unsure what to make of their results, but Robert Spitzer, who would later become the chairman for DSM-III, thought he knew both how to understand the problem of reliability, and, once he'd demonstrated a "crisis", also how to fix it. The statistical measure, Cohen's kappa, was key to Spitzer's argument (Spitzer, Cohen, Fleiss, & Endicott, 1967).

Cohen's kappa provides a measure of agreement that seeks to take into account that some level of agreement could be expected by chance. Cohen's kappa is defined as being $(p_o - p_c)/(1 - p_c)$ where p_o is the observed proportion of agreement and p_c the proportion expected by chance. A value of 0 indicates chance agreement; 1 indicates perfect agreement. At this point many readers' eyes will have glazed over. This glazing, Kirk and Kutchins (1992) point out in their history of the DSM-III, is important in understanding the evolution of debates about reliability in psychiatry. Cohen's kappa is a statistical innovation, but its utilisation complicated discussion of reliability to the extent where lay people and average clinicians could no longer contribute. While everyone may have a view as to whether it seems acceptable that a patient judged schizophrenic by one physician should have only a fifty per cent chance of being similarly diagnosed by a clinician giving a second opinion, who knows whether a kappa of 0.6 is acceptable?

Having introduced Cohen's kappa to psychiatrists, Spitzer (with co-author Joseph Fleiss, 1974) used it to reanalyse the existing reliability studies and to argue that the agreement achieved by clinicians using DSM-I and II was unacceptable. In their meta-analysis, Spitzer and Fleiss judged a kappa of over 0.7 to be "only satisfactory" (a level achieved only by diagnoses of mental deficiency, organic brain syndrome, and alcoholism), and condemned the kappas of less than 0.5 that were achieved by many of the diagnoses studied "poor". They conclude that "the reliability of psychiatric diagnosis as it has been practised since at least the late 1950s is not good" (Spitzer & Fleiss, 1974, p. 345). This judgment was echoed by later commentators. A key point for us is that in this paper Spitzer and Fleiss judged only values of Cohen's kappas greater than 0.7 to be satisfactory. Where had this threshold come from? No reference for it is provided in the paper. Kappa had not previously been employed in psychiatry and no conventional values for an acceptable kappa had been established. Spitzer and Fleiss were free to pick a threshold at their discretion.

When Spitzer became the chairman of the taskforce to develop DSM-III he continued to be concerned about the reliability of diagnosis. Field trials for the DSM-III included reliability tests. In these a Cohen's kappa of 0.7 continued to be the threshold for "good agreement" (APA, 1980, p. 468). For the most common diagnoses in adults—substance use disorders, schizophrenic disorders, and affective disorders—Cohen's kappas of 0.8 plus were reported. Spitzer and his colleagues were pleased, and concluded: "For adult patients, the reliability for most of the classes ... is quite good, and in general higher than that previously achieved with DSM-I and DSM-II" (APA, 1980, p. 468). Kirk and Kutchins provide a critique of the DSM-III field trials and a more modest assessment of their achievements. For us, however, the key question isn't whether the DSM-III truly was reliable, but that it was claimed to be—with reported kappas of 0.7 plus taken to be the proof.

When it came to the DSM-5, however, the goal posts seemed to shift. Prior to the results being available, members of the DSM-5 task force declared that a kappa of more than 0.8 would "be almost miraculous", a kappa between 0.6 and 0.8 would be "cause for celebration", values between 0.4 and 0.6 were a "realistic goal", and those between 0.2 and 0.4 "would be acceptable" (Kraemer, Kupfer, Clarke, Narrow, & Regier, 2012a). Data from a motley assortment of other reliability studies in medicine was cited to support the claim that such thresholds would be reasonable. These benchmarks were much lower than those employed in the DSM-III trials. Many commentators viewed these new standards as an attempt to soften up readers prior to the announcement of reliability results that, by historical standards, appeared shockingly poor (1 Boring Old Man, 2012; Frances, 2012b; Spitzer, Williams, & Endicott, 2012). Schizophrenia, which achieved a kappa of 0.81 in the DSM-III trial, had a kappa of 0.46 in the DSM-5 trial (Regier et al., 2013). Major affective disorders had a kappa of 0.8 with DSM-III and 0.28 with the DSM-5. Mixed anxiety-depressive disorder achieved a negative kappa—meaning that in this case clinicians would have been better off putting their diagnostic criteria in the bin and simply guessing. Of the twenty diagnoses studied in the DSM-5 field trial only three obtained kappas of more than 0.6.[1] Although commentators found the DSM-5 reliability results distinctly unimpressive, using their new thresholds for an acceptable kappa, the DSM-5 task force looked at their results and found that "most diagnoses adequately tested had good to very good reliability" (Regier et al., 2013, p. 59).

What should one make of these field trials? Were the results appalling, or good? Why were lower kappa scores obtained in the DSM-5 trials than in the DSM-III trials? And what threshold should one adopt for "acceptable" reliability?

First we can note that the methodology of the reliability studies had shifted, such that seeking to directly compare the DSM-III and DSM-5 trials is unfair. Many of the diagnoses studied in the DSM-5 field trial were new, and were generally at a "finer-grained level of resolution" than the diagnoses studied in the DSM-III trial. For example, while the DSM-III trial examined the reliability of "eating disorder" the DSM-5 trial looked at "binge eating". In the DSM-5 trial, clinicians independently interviewed the patients, at time intervals that ranged from four hours to two weeks. In the DSM-III trial, clinicians either jointly interviewed patients (but recorded their diagnoses separately) or interviewed them separately but as soon as possible. Such differences might partly account for the differing results.

Now for the shifting thresholds. While many psychiatrists have become used to thinking of Spitzer's threshold of 0.7 as the cut-off point for a "good" kappa, there are precedents for employing lower benchmarks in the statistical literature. Influentially, Landis and Koch (1977) count 0.21–0.4 fair, 0.41–0.6 moderate, 0.61–0.8 substantial, and 0.81 almost perfect. Altman (1991) condemns kappas of less than 0.2 poor, and considers anything above 0.61 good. Fleiss, Levin, and Cho Paik (2003) counts kappas below 0.4 poor, those between 0.4 and 0.75 fair to good, and those above 0.75 excellent. Clearly there are no universally agreed standards for what would count as a "good" Cohen's kappa.

In any case, I suggest that seeking some threshold for "acceptable" reliability to be applied across all contexts and all diagnoses is a mistake. Sometimes it is important for diagnosis to be very reliable; sometimes disagreements can be tolerated. In a research setting, it may matter a very great deal that the subject groups employed in different studies should be comparable. For research that depends on all subjects having the same disorder, the values of kappa that should be sought should be high. Sometimes the diagnosis that a patient receives is important because it makes a difference to the treatment that will be given. Mood stabilisers, such as lithium for example, are used only for bipolar disorders but not for other types of depression.

In many contexts, however, exacting standards of reliability need not be required. Suppose I am a marriage counsellor. My clients receive a DSM diagnosis that I place on their insurance forms, but I don't prescribe drugs; all my clients, regardless of diagnosis, receive exactly the same sort of talk-based therapy. In such a context, what does it matter if I diagnose a client as having a major depressive disorder while my colleague would have diagnosed them with an anxiety disorder? Even in drug-based therapy the link between diagnosis and drug type may not be tight. Many psychoactive medications are approved for the treatment of broad swathes of disorders and in such cases—so long as a wrong diagnosis makes no difference to treatment—little harm will be done.

The importance of achieving reliability varies with the diagnosis in question and with the context of use. When it makes little difference whether a particular diagnosis or those it is likely to be confused with gets made, "acceptable" kappas may be quite low. When there is a real risk that unreliable diagnosis will lead to harm, standards must be higher—either a higher value of kappa should be demanded or, if diagnostic criteria can't themselves be made reliable, mechanisms for dealing with uncertainty in practice may need to be employed (e.g., the routine use of second, or even third, opinions).

As we conclude, we are left with a puzzle. The point of the reliability tests was to demonstrate that the diagnostic criteria are reliable, but even now the results are in, it remains unclear whether the levels of reliability achieved are acceptable. This is because there are no generally accepted standards for what counts as reliable enough against which the DSM criteria can be judged.

With a different trial design, it might have been possible to at least show that progress had been made, and that the DSM-5 revisions produced criteria that could be applied more reliably than those in the DSM-IV. However, the shifts in methodology and statistics mean that the results of the DSM-5 field trial could never be directly compared with those of field trials for earlier DSMs. Changes in trial design were defended on the basis that methodology had improved: the DSM-III trials used the bad old ways, while the DSM-5 trials would use the new, good ways (e.g., Clarke et al., 2013; Kraemer, Kupfer, Clarke, Narrow, & Regier, 2012a). Fair enough. But then why was no head-to-head comparison of DSM-5 and DSM-IV criteria incorporated into the tests? (a possibility discussed by Ledford, 2012). The task force said head-to-head comparisons would make the trials too cumbersome, but in the absence of such tests, even now the DSM-5 field trial results are in, it is unclear whether or not the new system is more reliable than its predecessors.

Note

1. Current good practice is to give a 95% confidence interval when reporting values of kappa. I haven't done this here, as these were not recorded in the DSM-III study. If possible errors in kappa are taken into account in reporting the DSM-5 results, then the worst case estimates for these figures are even worse.

CHAPTER SEVEN

The future

Throughout this book I have shown how the DSM currently matters hugely. Even small changes can affect the lives of millions. In this last chapter, I look to the future. I shall explain why it is that I think the current dominance of the DSM is by no means guaranteed to continue. In looking ahead, the key point to bear in mind is that we should not assume that the DSM will long continue to exist in anything like its current form.

At the outset, it is worth noting that is likely that the DSM-5 will be the last time that the DSM comes to be revised all in one go and published in book form. The system for numbering volumes has been shifted to facilitate the publication of more regular smaller-scale revisions as and when needed. Rather than DSM-6 being published in 2030, we will have DSM 5.1, DSM 5.2, and maybe DSM 5.3.2.7 (Brauser, 2011; Verhoeff, 2010). This is all to the good. As mentioned previously, the current system meant that important copy editing errors in DSM-IV only came to be revised six years later. A process that allows for more frequent and easier updating can only be a good thing.

As well as the DSM coming to be updated more frequently, I expect more fundamental changes to occur. I think that the DSM will cease to be *the* classification of mental disorders used by researchers, clinicians, and service providers around the world, and will come to be just one classification amongst others. It is true that the DSM has been massively successful over the last three decades, but the grounds of this success are unstable. At present the DSM succeeds because it manages to be a good enough classification for multiple purposes. Crucially, at present, the DSM is employed by researchers, and the US medical insurance industry, and has also managed to maintain compatibility with the ICD. Use by researchers provides scientific credibility; entanglement with the mechanisms for insurance payment in the US ensures that the DSM sells enough copies to make money. At the same time, compatibility with the ICD makes the DSM system appear to be the only way of classifying mental disorders.

It is likely that over the next twenty years researchers in mental health will come to make less use of DSM categories. Many researchers have come to think that the sort of classification embodied in the DSM may not turn out to be the most fruitful for research. In 2009, the US National Institute of Mental Health launched its Research Domain Criteria project (RDoC) (NIMH, no date). This seeks to develop a new classification of psychopathology that may prove more useful for basic research. Crucially, the classifications included in RDoC will cut across traditional disorders. Instead of conducting research on panic disorder or schizophrenia, for example, researchers will instead do work on the problems that might affect the mechanisms that underpin fear or working memory.

Some within the APA have claimed that RDoC does not threaten the DSM (Insel & Lieberman, 2013). In their vision, if work using RDoC bears fruit then the DSM can be revised to reflect whatever new knowledge is gained. I think that if work using RDoC suggests a classification that differs much from the sorts of category that are currently included in the DSM, then radically revising the DSM to fit will prove difficult. As we have seen in the debates over the revisions to autism-related disorders proposed for the DSM-5, the entanglement of DSM categories with the mechanisms of service provision already means that even making relatively slight changes to the DSM has become very difficult.

A further difficulty would be that for the DSM to remain in widespread use, and to appear the only viable classification of mental disorders, it has to remain compatible with the ICD. However, the users and purposes of the ICD differ from those of the DSM (Reed, 2010). Currently the two classifications are broadly compatible, but if the DSM was altered to fit more closely the findings of basic science, there is no guarantee that the ICD would follow suit. The ICD comes in three versions. While the most complex is intended for use by researchers, two simplifications of this are produced—one for specialist clinicians, and one for use in primary care settings. Crucially all three versions of the ICD are intended to be compatible, and the WHO is committed to ensuring that the primary care version is suitable for use by non-specialist clinicians working in developing countries. This creates constraints on the possibilities for revising the ICD that might well limit the options for making the ICD more research focused.

Continued use by the US medical insurance industry is also important for the success of the DSM. The DSM is very expensive to produce (work on the DSM-5 cost $25 million (Frances, 2013, p. 175)). The APA is able to spend so much on the DSM because it makes even more through book sales, largely to mental health professionals who buy it in order to use the disorder codes for completing insurance forms. The APA puts a massive amount of work into ensuring that codes included in any new edition of the DSM are acceptable to the insurance industry but this acceptance is by no means guaranteed, especially if a new version differs greatly from its predecessor. The medical insurance industries can, if they choose, refuse to move to a new version of the DSM. Already at the time of writing, the US is one of the last countries on earth still to be using a version of

ICD-9 (the ICD-10 was published in 1990). The reason that the US has been so slow to move to the newer version of the ICD is that the systems used in funding US healthcare are so complex, and split between so many different powerful service providers, that forcing through changes to the codes on which they depend has become a monstrous undertaking (Reed, 2010). If the US medical insurance industry, and other bureaucratic systems, refused to move to a particular version of the DSM, then sales of the DSM would plummet.

The success of the DSM has also been linked with the fact that the US has been the largest market for pharmaceuticals. As a result, companies developing and marketing new drugs have concentrated on satisfying regulators and clinicians in the US. And, in the US, regulators and clinicians have become used to psychoactive drugs being aimed at DSM diagnoses. Most notably, the FDA demands that clinical trials show that drugs are effective before they will be approved, and in the case of psycho-pharmaceuticals the clinical trials submitted to the FDA have tended to make use of DSM categories to select subject populations. At some point, however, the US may well cease to be the largest market for psychoactive pharmaceuticals. China, for example, has a rapidly expanding economy and a massive population. If China became a more important market for pharmaceuticals than the US, then rather than pharmaceutical companies courting the US market, and so using the DSM, they would instead prioritise research and marketing that was acceptable to Chinese regulators and buyers. The consequences are hard to predict, but maybe a Chinese market would come to favour studies couched in the terms of locally developed classifications, such as the ICD-Chinese modification. In such a case the dominance of the DSM would be undermined.

Considering all these factors together, we can see that current support of the DSM is brittle. In the future it is likely that at least one key user group—researchers, the insurance industry, or the pharmaceutical industry—will at least partially switch to an alternative classification. The ICD may also come to diverge from the DSM. In any such scenario, the DSM might well continue, but would become one amongst a number of classification systems, each used for different purposes.

Having a diversity of classifications of mental health issues for different purposes would in many ways be an improvement. The most striking thing about the DSM-5 is how very similar it is to the DSM-IV. Plausibly this is largely because the DSM currently seeks to satisfy so many different constituencies that making any changes to it is very difficult. Changes that researchers may want, for example, can prove impossible if they turn out to be unacceptable to service providers, or to the developers of the ICD. If the DSM had to keep fewer groups happy, then it would be freer to make revisions.

Having distinct classifications for distinct purposes—research and determining service provision, say—would be a good thing. Even if we just think about the needs of researchers, it is plausible that multiple classifications might be useful. The philosopher John Dupré has argued for a view he calls "promiscuous realism" (Dupré, 1981, 1993). The basic idea is that the world is such that very many potentially fruitful classifications are possible. Dupré points out that different researchers in biology find different ways of classifying species useful (Dupré, 2001). Ecologists are most interested in the current characteristics of organisms, and for such purposes distinguishing species on the basis of current characteristics makes sense. Evolutionary theorists, on the other hand, pose research questions that are best served by a classification that depends on relations of ancestry. Dupré argues that all can live in harmony, and that particular sub-disciplines should be permitted to classify as best suits their needs. I expect that multiple classifications might also be useful for research in mental health. Ken Kendler takes the case of schizophrenia, and discusses evidence that the criteria that pick out subtypes that best predict treatment response may be different from those that best fit with familial aggregation (Kendler, 1990). Depending of the research question, different ways of splitting up the schizophrenias will be most useful.

Having multiple classifications might also help avoid current problems that emerge when the DSM—a classification developed largely for US populations—comes to be employed around the world. I see two main problems with the DSM being used worldwide. First, and this has been widely noted, the ways in which mental distress are manifested plausibly differ cross-culturally (e.g., Mellsop et al., 2011). At present the disorders of non-US populations risk being shoe-horned into US categories. Second, there is currently a tension between the guideline that revisions to the DSM should do more good than harm (discussed in Chapter Four) and the idea that the DSM should be used globally. In weighing harms and benefits, the DSM committees seek to assess factors such as how likely it is that a diagnosis will lead to the harmful treatment of false positives; how likely it is that diagnosis will lead to helpful early intervention; and how likely is it that diagnosis will lead to particular groups being stigmatised. However, the answers to such questions are highly context sensitive; the impact of a diagnosis of alcohol use disorder, for example, will likely be very different for someone in the US as compared to Pakistan. Whether a new diagnosis will do more good than harm depends on where that diagnosis is likely to be made. As such, any classification that seeks to do more good than harm is best intended for use in specific and circumscribed contexts rather than universally. In the future I expect the DSM to be less important. The current situation—with one classification system being used by all researchers, by clinicians, and in determining service provision—will not continue. The DSM will become just one amongst others, bringing hope that a multiplicity of classifications will help improve mental health research and care.

REFERENCES

1 Boring Old Man. (2012). *To take us seriously.* Posted 22 May 2012. Available at http://1boringoldman.com/index.php/2012/05/22/to-take-us-seriously/ [last accessed 21 July 2013].

Altman, D. (1991). *Practical Statistics for Medical Research.* London: Chapman and Hall.

American Psychiatric Association. (1952). *Diagnostic and Statistical Manual: Mental Disorders.* Washington, DC: American Psychiatric Association.

American Psychiatric Association. (1968). *Diagnostic and Statistical Manual of Mental Disorders. (2nd edition).* Washington, DC: American Psychiatric Association.

American Psychiatric Association. (1980). *Diagnostic and Statistical Manual of Mental Disorders (3rd edn).* Washington, DC: American Psychiatric Association.

American Psychiatric Association. (1987). *Diagnostic and Statistical Manual of Mental Disorders. (3rd edn, revised).* Washington, DC: American Psychiatric Association.

American Psychiatric Association. (1993). *DSM-IV Draft Criteria.* Washington, DC: American Psychiatric Association.

American Psychiatric Association. (1994). *Diagnostic and Statistical Manual of Mental Disorders (4th edn).* Washington, DC: American Psychiatric Association.

REFERENCES

American Psychiatric Association. (2000). *Diagnostic and Statistical Manual of Mental Disorders* (4th edn, text revision). Washington, DC: American Psychiatric Association.

American Psychiatric Association. (2005). 2005 annual report. Available at www.psychiatry.org/about-apa--psychiatry/annual-reports [Last accessed 21 July 2013].

American Psychiatric Association. (2011). Protocol for DSM-5 field trials in routine clinical practice settings. Dated 18 March 2011. Available at www.dsm5.org/Research/Documents/DSM5%20FT%20RCP%20Protocol%2003–19–11%20revlc.pdf [Last accessed 21 July 2013].

American Psychiatric Association. (2012a). Treasurer's report. May 2012. Available at https://docs.google.com/file/d/0BzWdENl1wkVSYk5aXzRZelFYUjA/edit?pli=1 [Last accessed 21 July 2013].

American Psychiatric Association. (2012b). Reports to the membership. *American Journal of Psychiatry, 169*: 999–1004.

American Psychiatric Association. (2013). *Diagnostic and Statistical Manual of Mental Disorders.* (5th edn). Washington, DC: American Psychiatric Association.

American Psychiatric Association. (no date). DSM-5 in Development. Board of Trustee Principles. Available at www.dsm5.org/about/Pages/BoardofTrusteePrinciples.aspx [Last accessed 21 July 2013].

Axelson, D., Birmaher, B., Findling, R., Fristad, M., Kowatch, R., Youngstrom, E., Arnold, L., Goldstein, B., Goldstein, T., Chang, K., DelBello, M., Ryan N., & Diler, R. (2011). Concerns regarding the inclusion of temper dysregulation disorder with dysphoria in the *Diagnostic and Statistical Manual of Mental Disorders*, Fifth Edition. *Journal of Clinical Psychiatry, 72*: 1257–1262.

Bayer, R. (1981). *Homosexuality and American Psychiatry*. New York: Basic Books.

Board of Trustees. (2007). DSM-V task force and work group acceptance form. Amended and approved by BOT October 2007. Available at www.dsm5.org/about/Documents/DSM%20Member%20 Acceptance%20Form.pdf [Last accessed 21 July 2013].

Brauser, D. (2011). APA answers DSM-5 critics. Nov 9. Medscape Medical News. Available at www.medscape.com/viewarticle/753255 [Last accessed 26 July 2013].

Caplan, P. (1995). *They Say You're Crazy: How the World's Most Powerful Psychiatrists Decide Who's Normal*. Reading, MA: Addison-Wesley.

Caplan, P. (2008). Pathologizing your period. *Ms*. Summer 2008: 63–64.

Caplan, P. (2011). What? Psychiatrists now define "openness"? (Part 2). Posted on 4 May 2011 in Science Isn't Golden. Blog on Psychology Today. Available at www.psychologytoday.com/blog/science-isnt-golden/201105/what-psychiatrists-now-define-openness-part-2 [Last accessed 21 July 2013].

Cassels, C. (2010). New code of conduct formalizes APA's relationship with the pharmaceutical industry. June 28 2010. *Medscape Medical News*. Available at www.medscape.com/viewarticle/724255 [Last accessed 21 July 2013].

Chapman, S. (2012). DSM-5 SSD submissions 2012. On dx revision watch blog. Available at http://dxrevisionwatch.com/dsm-5-drafts/dsm-5-ssd-submissions-2012 [Last accessed 21 July 2013].

Chapman, S. (no date). Dx revision watch. About. Available at http://dxrevisionwatch.com/about/ [Last accessed 21 July 2013].

Clarke, D., Narrow, W., Regier, D., Kuramoto, S., Kupfer, D., Kuhl, E., Greiner, L., & Kraemer, H. (2013). DSM-5 field trials in the United States and in Canada, Part 1: Study design, sampling strategy, implementation, and analytic approaches. *American Journal of Psychiatry, 170*: 43–58.

Cobb, A. (1996). *Mind's Yellow Card Scheme Reporting the Adverse Effects of Psychiatric Drugs. First report*. May 1996. London: Mind.

Cobb, A., Darton, K., & Juttla, K. (2001). *Mind's Yellow Card for Reporting Drug Side Effects: A Report of Users' Experiences*. London: Mind.

Conrad, P. (2007). *The Medicalization of Society*. Baltimore, MD: Johns Hopkins University Press.

Cooper, R. (2007). *Psychiatry and Philosophy of Science*. Stocksfield: Acumen.

Cooper, R. (2012). Is psychiatric classification a good thing? In: K. Kendler & J. Parnas (Eds.), *Philosophical Issues in Psychiatry II: Nosology* (pp. 61–70). Oxford: Oxford University Press.

Cosgrove, L., & Krimsky, S. (2012). A comparison of *DSM-IV* and *DSM-5* panel members' financial associations with industry: A pernicious problem persists. *PLoS Medicine 9*(3): e1001190.

Davies, J. (2012). Label jars, not people: Lobbying against the shrinks. *New Scientist, 2865*(17 May 2012): 7.

Denton, W. (2007). Issues for DSM-V: Relational diagnosis: An essential component of biopsychosocial assessment. *American Journal of Psychiatry, 164*: 1146–1147.

Dickerson Mayes, S., Black, A., & Tierney, C. (2013). DSM-5 underidentifies PDDNOS: Diagnostic agreement between the DSM-5, DSM-IV, and checklist for autism spectrum disorder. *Research in Autism Spectrum Disorders, 7*: 298–306.

Dupré, J. (1981). Natural kinds and biological taxa. *The Philosophical Review, XC*: 66–90.

Dupré, J. (1993). *The Disorder of Things*. Cambridge, MA: Harvard University Press.

Dupré, J. (2001). In defence of classification. *Studies in History and Philosophy of Biological and Biomedical Sciences, 32*: 203–219.

Edwards, J. (2009). Pfizer turned NAMI into "Trojan horse" to push Geodon off-label to kids, suit claims. *CBS News Moneywatch*. 16 September 2009, available at http://www.cbsnews.com/news/pfizer-turned-nami-into-trojan-horse-to-push-geodon-off-label-to-kids-suit-claims/ [Last accessed 13 Jan 2014].

Fachner, J. (2006). An ethno-methodological approach to cannabis and music perception, with EEG brain mapping in a naturalistic setting. *Anthropology of Consciousness, 17*: 78–103.

First, M. (2009). Harmonisation of ICD-11 and DSM-V: opportunities and challenges. *The British Journal of Psychiatry, 195*: 382–390.

First, M., & Pincus, H. (2002). The DSM-IV Text Revision: Rationale and potential impact on clinical practice. *Psychiatric Services, 53*: 288–292.

Fleiss, J., Levin, B., & Cho Paik, M. (2003). *Statistical Methods for Rates and Proportions (3rd edn)*. New York: John Wiley.

Frances, A. (2012a). Is DSM-5 a public trust or an APA cash cow? Commercialism and censorship trump concern for quality. In DSM in Distress blog on Psychology Today. Posted 3 January 2012. Available at www.psychologytoday.com/blog/dsm5-in-distress/201201/is-dsm-5-public-trust-or-apa-cash-cow [Last accessed 21 July 2013].

Frances, A. (2012b). DSM-5 field trials discredit the American Psychiatric Association. Huffington Post Science. The Blog. Posted 31 October 2012. Available at www.huffingtonpost.com/allen-frances/dsm-5-field-trials-discre_b_2047621.html [Last accessed 21 July 2013].

Frances, A. (2013). *Saving Normal*. New York: Harper Collins.

Friedman, R. (2012). Grief, depression and the DSM-5. *New England Journal of Medicine, 366*: 1855–1857.

Frost, R., & Hartl, T. (1996). A cognitive-behavioral model of compulsive hoarding. *Behaviour Research and Therapy, 34*: 341–350.

Frost, R., Ruby, D., Shuer, L. (2012). The buried in treasures workshop: Waitlist control trial of facilitated support groups for hoarding. *Behaviour Research and Therapy, 50*: 661–667.

Gembris, H. (Ed.) (2006). *Musical Development from a Lifespan Perspective*. Frankfurt am Main: Peter Lang.

Ghaemi, N., Bauer, M., Cassidy, F., Malhi, G., Mitchell, P., Phelps, J., Vieta, E., Youngstrom, E., & for the ISBD Diagnostic Guidelines Task Force (2008). Diagnostic guidelines for bipolar disorder: A summary of the *International Society for Bipolar Disorders* Diagnostic Guidelines Task Force Report. *Bipolar Disorders, 10*: 117–128.

Government Accountability Office (2006). Federal autism activities: Funding for research has increased, but agencies need to resolve surveillance challenges. Report GAO-06–700. 19 July 2006. United States Government Accountability Office.

Greenberg, G. (2013). *The Book of Woe: The DSM and the Unmaking of Psychiatry*. New York: Blue Rider.

Happé, F. (2011). Criteria, categories, and continua: autism and related disorders in *DSM-5*. *Journal of the American Academy of Child and Adolescent Psychiatry, 50*: 540–542.

Haraway, D. (1989). *Primate Visions: Gender, Race, and Nature in the World of Modern Science*. London: Routledge.

Harmon, A. (2012). A specialists' debate on autism has many worried observers. *The New York Times* (New York edn), 21 January, p. A13.

Harris, G. (2008). Research center tied to drug company. *The New York Times* (New York edn), 25 November, p. A22.

Harris, G. (2009). Drug maker told studies would aid it, papers say. *The New York Times* (New York edn), 19 March, p. A16.

Healy, D. (1997). *The Antidepressant Era*. Cambridge, MA: Harvard University Press.

Healy, D. (2006). Did regulators fail over selective serotonin reuptake inhibitors? *British Medical Journal, 333*: 92–95.

Heisel, W. (2012). Slap: American Psychiatric Association pressures Brit DSM-5 blogger Suzy Chapman. Blog William Heisel's Antidote: Investigating Untold Health Stories. Posted 27 February. Available at www.reportingonhealth.org/blogs/2012/02/27/slap-american-psychiatric-association-pressures-brit-dsm5-blogger-suzy-chapman. [Last accessed 21 July 2013].

Huerta, M., Bishop, S., Duncan, A., Hus, V., & Lord, C. (2012). Application of DSM-5 criteria for autism spectrum disorder to three samples of children with DSM-IV diagnoses of pervasive developmental disorders. *American Journal of Psychiatry, 169*: 1056–1064.

In-cites (2007). The most-cited researchers in psychiatry/psychology. Available at http://in-cites.com/top/2007/second07-psy.html [Last accessed 21 July 2013].

Insel, T., & Lieberman, J. (2013). DSM-5 and RDoC: Shared interests. Press release May 13. NIMH website. Available at www.nimh.nih.gov/news/science-news/2013/dsm-5-and-rdoc-shared-interests.shtml [Last accessed 27 July 2013].

Kaplan, A. (2008). Senate investigations spread to APA and ACCME. *Psychiatric Times*, 1 September. Available at http://www.psychiatrictimes.com/senate-investigations-spread-apa-and-accme [Last accessed 21 July 2013].

Kaslow, F. (1993). Relational diagnosis: An idea whose time has come? *Family Process, 32*: 255–259.

Kendler, K. (1990). Toward a scientific psychiatric nosology: Strengths and limitations. *Archives of General Psychiatry, 47*: 969–973.

Kendler, K., Kupfer, D., Narrow, W., Phillips, K., & Fawcett, J. (2009). Guidelines for making changes to DSM-V. Revised 21.10.09. Available at www.dsm5.org/ProgressReports/Documents/Guidelines-for-Making-Changes-to-DSM_1.pdf [Last accessed 23 July 2013].

Kirk, S., & Kutchins, H. (1992). *The Selling of DSM: The Rhetoric of Science in Psychiatry*. New York: Aldine de Gruyter.

Kluger, B., Cacciatore, J., & Montgomery, K. (2012). Revolution on standby: bereavement and the DSM-5. Letter on behalf of MISS to the APA. Dated 31 October. Available at http://drjoanne.blogspot.co.uk/2012/10/revolution-on-standby.html [Last accessed 21 July 2013].

Knudson, G., De Cuypere, G., & Bockting, W. (2010). Process toward consensus of the recommendations for revision of the DSM diagnoses of gender identity disorders by the World Professional Association for Transgender Health. *International Journal of Transgenderism, 12*: 54–59.

Kraemer, H., Kupfer, D., Clarke, D., Narrow, W., & Regier, D. (2012a). DSM-5: How reliable is reliable enough? *American Journal of Psychiatry, 169*: 13–15.

Kraemer, H., Kupfer, D., Clarke, D., Narrow, W., & Regier, D. (2012b). Response to Spitzer et al Letter. *American Journal of Psychiatry, 169*: 537–538.

Kupfer, D. (2012). DSM field trials providing ample critical data. *Psychiatric News, 47*: 1a–28.

Kupfer, D., First, M., & Regier, D. (Eds.) (2002). *A Research Agenda for DSM-V*. Washington, DC: American Psychiatric Association.

Kushner, H. (1999). *A Cursing Brain? The Histories of Tourette Syndrome*. Cambridge, MA: Harvard University Press.

Kushner, H. (2004). Competing medical cultures, support groups, and Tourette syndrome. In: R. Packard, P. Brown, R. Berkelman, & H. Frumkin (Eds.), *Emerging Illness and Society: Negotiating the Public Health Agenda* (pp. 71–101). Baltimore, MD: Johns Hopkins University Press.

Lancet (2012). Living with grief: Editorial. *The Lancet, 379*: 589.

Landis, J., & Koch, G. (1977). The measurement of observer agreement for categorical data. *Biometrics, 33*: 159–174.

LeBeau, R., Glenn, D., Liao, B., Wittchen, H., Beesdo-Baum, K., Ollendick, T., & Craske, M. (2010). Specific phobia: a review of DSM-IV specific phobia and preliminary recommendations for DSM-V. *Depression and Anxiety*, 27: 148–167.

Ledford, H. (2012). DSM field trials inflame debate over psychiatric testing. Nature News Blog. Posted 5 November. Available at http://blogs.nature.com/news/2012/11/dsm-field-trials-inflame-debate-over-psychiatric-testing.html [Last accessed 21 July 2013].

Leonard, H., Dixon, G., Whitehouse, A., Bourke, J., Aiberti, K., Nassar, N., Bower, C., & Glasson, E. (2010). Unpacking the complex nature of the autism epidemic. *Research in Autism Spectrum Disorders*, 4: 548–554.

Lewis, B. (2012). Reflections on the 2012 radical caucus meeting. Mad in America. 8 May. Available at www.madinamerica.com/2012/05/op-ed-5/ [Last accessed 21 July 2013].

Liu, K., King, M., & Bearman, P. (2010). Social influence and the autism epidemic. *American Journal of Sociology*, 115: 1387–1434.

Longino, H. (1990). *Science as Social Knowledge: Values and Objectivity in Scientific Inquiry*. Princeton, NJ: Princeton University Press.

Lord, C., Petkova, E., Hus, V., Gan, W., Lu, F., Martin, D., Ousley, O., Guy, L., Bernier, R., Gerdts, J., Algermissen, M., Whitaker, A., Sutcliffe, J., Warren, Z., Klin, A., Saulnier, C., Hanson, E., Hundley, R., Piggot, J., Fombonne, E., Steiman, M., Miles, J., Kanne, S., Goin-Kochel, R., Peters, S., Cook, E., Guter, S., Tjernagel, J., Green-Snyder, L., Bishop, S., Esler, A., Gotham, K., Luyster, R., Miller, F., Olson, J., Richler, J., & Risi, S. (2012). A multisite study of the clinical diagnosis of different autism spectrum disorders. *Archives of General Psychiatry*, 69: 306–313.

Martin, L. (2012). APA rebuts study of autism. *Psychiatric Times*. 30 March. Available at www.psychiatrictimes.com/autism/apa-rebuts-study-autism [Last accessed 21 July 2013].

Mataix-Cols, D. (no date). Hoarding disorder: what it is, and what it is not. Help for Hoarders website. Available at www.helpforhoarders.co.uk/what-is-hoarding/ [Last accessed 21 July 2013].

Mataix-Cols, D., Billotti, D., Fernández de la Cruz, L., & Nordsletten, A. (2013). The London field trial for hoarding disorder. *Psychological Medicine, 43*: 837–847.

Mataix-Cols, D., Frost, R., Pertusa, A., Clark, L., Saxena, S., Leckman, J., Stein, D., Matsunaga, H., & Wilhelm, S. (2010). Hoarding disorder: A new diagnosis for DSM-V? *Depression and Anxiety, 27*: 556–572.

Mather, C. (2005). The pipeline and the porcupine: alternate metaphors of the physician-industry relationship. *Social Science and Medicine, 60*: 1323–1334.

Matson, J., & Wilkins, J. (2008). Nosology and diagnosis in Asperger's syndrome. *Research in Autism Spectrum Disorders, 2*: 288–300.

Matson, J., Belva, B., Horovitz, M., Kozlowski, A., & Bamburg, J. (2012). Comparing symptoms of autism spectrum disorders in a developmentally disabled adult population using the current *DSM-IV-TR* diagnostic criteria and the proposed *DSM-5* diagnostic criteria. *Journal of Developmental and Physical Disabilities, 24*: 403–414.

Mattila, M., Kielinen, M., Linna, S., Jussila, K., Ebeling, H., Bloigu, R., Joseph, R., & Moilanen, I. (2011). Autism spectrum disorders according to *DSM-IV-TR* and comparison with *DSM-5* draft criteria: An epidemiological study. *Journal of the American Academy of Child and Adolescent Psychiatry, 50*: 583–592.e11.

McCleary, K. (2010). Letter to the DSM-5 task force from the CFIDS association of America. Available at www.cfids.org/advocacy/2010/dsm5-statement.pdf [Last accessed 21 July 2013].

Mellsop, G., Janca, A., León-Andrade, C., Nga Yan Luk, D., Fung Kum Chiu, H., Elder, H., Shinfuku, N., Tapsell, R., Balaratnasingam, S., & Chi Chan, W. (2011). Asian/Pacific Rim psychiatrists' views on aspects of future classifications. *Asia-Pacific Psychiatry, 3*: 228–234.

Moran, M. (2009). DSM-V developers weigh adding psychosis risk. *Psychiatric News, August 21, 44*: (16)5.

Moreno, C., Laje, G., Blanco, C., Jiang, H., Schmidt, A., & Olfson, M. (2007). National trends in the outpatient diagnosis and treatment of bipolar disorder in youth. *Archives of General Psychiatry, 64*: 1032–1039.

Mościcki, E., Clarke, D., Kuramoto, S., Kraemer, H., Narrow, W., Kupfer, D., & Regier, D. (2013). Testing *DSM-5* in routine clinical practice settings: feasibility and clinical utility. *Psychiatric Services, 64*: 952–960.

National Institute of Mental Health (no date). Research Domain Criteria (RDoc) National Institute of Mental Health website. Available at www.nimh.nih.gov/research-priorities/rdoc/index.shtml [Last accessed 21 July 2013].

Ne'eman, A., & Kapp, S. (2012). What are the stakes? An analysis of the impact of the DSM-5 draft autism criteria on law, policy and service provision. June 2012. Autistic Self Advocacy Network. Available at http://autisticadvocacy.org/wp-content/uploads/2012/06/DSM-5_Policy_Brief_ASAN_final.pdf [Last accessed 21 July 2013].

Oldham, J. (2011). Letter from John Oldham, President American Psychiatric Association to Don Locke, President American Counselling Association dated 21 November 2011. Available at www.psychiatrictimes.com/all/editorial/psychiatrictimes/pdfs/apa-response-aca.pdf [Last accessed 21 July 2013].

Parens, E., & Johnston, J. (2010). Controversies concerning the diagnosis and treatment of bipolar disorder in children. *Child and Adolescent Psychiatry and Mental Health, 4*: 9.

Peele, P., Lave, J., & Kelleher, K. (2002). Exclusions and limitations in children's behavioural health care coverage. *Psychiatric Services, 53*: 591–594.

Phillips, J. (2010). Another DSM on the shelf? *Association for the Advancement of Philosophy and Psychiatry Bulletin, 17*: (2)70–71. Available at http://alien.dowling.edu/~cperring/aapp/bulletin_v_17_2/Vol17N2.pdf [Last accessed 5 November 2013].

Pinborough-Zimmerman, J., Bakian, A., Fombonne, E., Bilder, D., Taylor, J., & McMahon, W. (2012). Changes in the administrative prevalence of autism spectrum disorders: Contribution of special education and health from 2002–2008. *Journal of Autism and Developmental Disorders, 42*: 521–530.

Psychiatric News (1980). News and notes. *Psychiatric News*, 15 February, p. 11.

Pulli, K., Karma, K., Norio, R., Sistonen, P., Göring, H., & Järvelä, I. (2008). Genome-wide linkage scan for loci of musical aptitude in Finnish families: evidence for a major locus at 4q22. *Journal of Medical Genetics*, 45: 451–456.

Ramsay, J., & Waite, R. (no date). ADHD diagnosis for DSM-5; ADDA comments on proposed changes to the diagnostic manual. Available at www.add.org/?page=DSM5 [Last accessed 21 July 2013].

Reed, G. (2010). Toward ICD-11: Improving the clinical utility of WHO's International Classification of Mental Disorders. *Professional Psychology: Research and Practice*, 41: 457–464.

Regier, D., Kuhl, E., Kupfer, D., & McNulty, J. (2010). Patient involvement in the development of DSM-V. *Psychiatry: Interpersonal and Biological Processes*, 73: 308–310.

Regier, D., Narrow, W., Clarke, D., Kraemer, H., Kuramoto, S., Kuhl, E., & Kupfer, D. (2013). DSM-5 field trials in the United States and Canada, Part II: Test-retest reliability of selected categorical diagnoses. *American Journal of Psychiatry*, 170: 59–70.

Schlaug, G. (2003). The brain of musicians. In: I. Peretz & R. Zattore (Eds.) *The Cognitive Neuroscience of Music*, (pp. 366–381). Oxford: Oxford University Press.

Siklos, S., & Kerns, K. (2007). Assessing the diagnostic experiences of a small sample of parents of children with autism spectrum disorders. *Research in Developmental Disabilities*, 28: 9–22.

Singer, E. (2012). Diagnosis: Redefining autism. *Nature*, 491: S12–S13.

Spitzer, R. (2004). Good idea or politically correct nonsense? *Psychiatric Services*, 55: 113.

Spitzer, R., & Fleiss, J. (1974). A re-analysis of the reliability of psychiatric diagnosis. *British Journal of Psychiatry*, 125: 341–347.

Spitzer, R., Williams, J., & Endicott, J. (2012). Standards for DSM-5 reliability. Letters to the editor. *American Journal of Psychiatry*, 169: 537.

Spitzer, R., Cohen, J., Fleiss, J., & Endicott, J. (1967). Quantification of agreement in psychiatric diagnosis. *Archives of General Psychiatry*, 17: 83–87.

Strasser, S. (1999). *Waste and Want: A Social History of Trash*. New York: Henry Holt.
The Conversation (2012). What does a hoarder's brain look like? Study calls for rethink on treatment. Available at http://theconversation.com/what-does-a-hoarders-brain-look-like-study-calls-for-rethink-on-treatment-8705 [Last accessed 21 July 2013].
Verhoeff, B. (2010). Drawing borders of mental disorders: an interview with David Kupfer. *BioSocieties, 5*: 467–475.
Volkmar, F. (1992). Childhood disintegrative disorder: issues for DSM-IV. *Journal of Autism and Developmental Disorders, 22*: 625–642.
Volkmar, F., Klin, A., Siegel, B., Szatmari, P., Lord, C., Campbell, M., Freeman, B., Cicchetti, D., Rutter, M., Kline, W., Buitelaar, J., Hattab, Y., Fombonne, E., Fuentes, J., Werry, J., Stone, W., Kerbeshian, J., Hoshino, Y., Bregman, J., Loveland, K., Szymanski, L., & Towbin, K. (1994). Field trial for autistic disorder in DSM-IV. *American Journal of Psychiatry, 151*: 1361–1367.
Whoriskey, P. (2012). Antidepressants to treat grief? Psychiatry panelists with ties to drug industry say yes. *Washington Post*, 26 December. Available at http://articles.washingtonpost.com/2012-12-26/business/36015527_1_drug-companies-antidepressants-wellbutrin [Last accessed 21 July 2013].
Wieczner, J. (2013). Drug companies look to profit from DSM-5. Binge eating and hoarding diagnoses may lead to new sales. MarketWatch, The Wall Street Journal, 5 June. Available at www.marketwatch.com/story/new-psych-manual-could-create-drug-windfalls-2013-06-05 [Last accessed 21 July 2013].
Williams, K., Tuck, M., Helmer, M., Bartak, L., Mellis, C., & Peat, J. on behalf of the Autism Spectrum Disorder Steering Group (2008). Diagnostic labelling of autism spectrum disorders in NSW. *Journal of Paediatrics and Child Health, 44*: 108–113.
Young, A. (1995). *The Harmony of Illusions: Inventing Post-Traumatic Stress Disorder*. Princeton, NJ: Princeton University Press.

INDEX

1 Boring Old Man 50, 52

Altman, D. 53
American Psychiatric
 Association ix–xi, xiii, 13–14,
 21–27, 45–46, 58
anxiety disorders 5, 16, 52, 54
appendix, of conditions for
 further study 5–6
Asperger's disorder 9–10, 40–43,
 45–46
attention-deficit/hyperactivity
 disorder xii, 4, 7
attenuated psychosis
 syndrome 6
autism 9–10, 40–48
Autistic Self Advocacy Network
 45
autistic spectrum disorder 9–10,
 40–48
Axelson, D. 18

Bamburg, J. 41
Bayer, R. xiii, 22

Bearman, P. 43–44
Belva, B. 41
bereavement xiii, 7
Biederman, J. 17
Billotti, D. 38
binge eating 6–7
bipolar disorder 16–19
Bishop, S. 42
Black, A. 41
Board of Trustees xiii
Bockting, W. xii–xiii
body dysmorphic disorder 11
Brauser, D. 30 n.1, 64
bulimia nervosa 7

Cacciatore, J. xiii
Caplan, P. xiii, 12 n.1, 6, 26
Cassels, C. 14
Chapman, S. 24, 26
childhood disintegrative
 disorder 10
China 59
Cho Paik, M. 53
chronic fatigue syndrome xii, 24

Clarke, D. 42, 52, 55
clinical significance criterion x, 8, 11
Cobb, A. 28
cognitive behavioural therapy 39
Cohen, J. 50
Cohen's kappa *see* kappa
Conrad, P. 4
consultation, DSM-5 web xi, 23–26
Cooper, R. xvi n.2, 28
copy editing, problems in DSM 12 n.3, 46
Cosgrove, L. 14
cost, DSM-5 xi
cross-cultural 61

Darton, K. 28
Davies, J. xiv, 22
De Cuypere, G. xii–xiii
Denton, W. xii
depression ix, 7, 15–16, 19, 54
Dickerson Mayes, S. 41
dimensional classification 3
disorder, DSM definition 34
disruptive mood dysregulation disorder 12 n.3, 16–18
dissociative identity disorder 11
distress or impairment, DSM criterion of x, 8, 11, 32, 35
DSM-I xi, 51
DSM-II xi, 51
DSM-III xi–xii, 2, 6, 34, 49–53
DSM-III-R xi, 5–6
DSM-IV xi, xiv, xvi n.1, 3, 6–7, 9, 32, 40–41, 46–47, 60

DSM-IV-TR xi, 3, 7–8, 34, 46–47
Duncan, A. 42
Dupré, J. 60

Edwards, J. 19–20 n.1
Endicott, J. 50, 52–53
excoriation (skin picking) 6

Fachner, J. 37
family therapy xii, 39
Fawcett, J. 14, 35
FDA *see* Food and Drug Administration
Fernández de la Cruz, L. 38
field trials 26, 30 n.1, 42, 49–55
First, M. x, xvi n.1, 1–2, 47
Fleiss, J. 50–51, 53
Food and Drug Administration (FDA) 20 n.1, 59
Frances, A. xi, 7–9, 23, 50, 52, 58
Friedman, R. 7
Frost, R. 31–33, 39

Gembris, H. 37
Ghaemi, N. 17
gift relationship 15
Greenberg, G. 7, 11, 46
grief xiii, 7

Happé, F. 41, 45
Haraway, D. 28
Harmon, A. 45
Harris, G. 17
Hartl, T. 31–33
Healy, D. 15–16, 28
Heisel, W. 26
hoarding disorder 6, 29, 31–39

homosexuality xiii, 22
Horovitz, M. 41
Huerta, M. 42
Hus, V. 42

In-cites 17
Insel, T. 57
insomnia disorder 11
insurance x, 44, 57–58
intellectual disability 43–44
International Classification of Diseases (ICD) x–xi, xvi n.1, 21, 57–59
International OCD Foundation 32
internet use gaming disorder 6

Johnson and Johnson 17
Johnston, J. 16
junk 36–37
Juttla, K. 28

Kaplan, A. 13–14
Kapp, S. 45
kappa 50–54, 55 n.1
Kaslow, F. xii
Kelleher, K. 44
Kendler, K. 35, 60–61
Kerns, K. 43
King, M. 43–44
Kirk, S. 50–52
Kluger, B. xiii
Knudson, G. xii–xiii
Koch, G. 53
Kozlowski, A. 41
Kraemer, H. 52, 55
Krimsky, S. 14

Kuhl, E. 23
Kupfer, D. xi, 1–2, 23, 30 n.1, 35, 45, 52, 55
Kushner, H. xii
Kutchins, H. 50–52

Lancet 7
Landis, J. 53
Lave, J. 44
LeBeau, R. 8
Leonard, H. 43
Levin, B. 53
Lewis, B. 23
Lieberman, J. 57
Liu, K. 43–44
Longino, H. 28
Lord, C. 41–42

Martin, L. 45
Mataix-Cols, D. 33, 35, 38
Mather, C. 15
Matson, J. 40–41
Mattila, M. 41
McCleary, K. xii
McNulty, J. 23
ME (myalgic encephalomyelitis) *see* chronic fatigue syndrome
Medicaid 48
medicalisation 4, 38
Mellsop, G. 61
menstrual cycle mood variations xiii, 6, 12
MIND 19, 28–29
Mindfreedom 23
mixed anxiety-depressive disorder 52
Montgomery, K. xiii

Moran, M. 6
Moreno, C. 16–17
Mościcki, E. 30 n.1
multiple personality disorder 11
musical ability 37

Narrow, W. 35, 52, 55
National Alliance on Mental Illness (NAMI) 19 n.1, 23
National Institute of Mental Health (NIMH) 57
Ne'eman, A. 45
Nordsletten, A. 38
not otherwise specified (NOS) codes 5, 11, 18–19, 39–40, 46

Oaks, D. 23
Obsessive-compulsive disorder (OCD) 16, 32–34
obsessive-compulsive personality disorder 6, 31
Oldham, J. 22
"other" codes 5, 11, 18–19, 39

panic disorder 16
paraphilia 7–8
Parens, E. 16
patients
 patient groups xii–xiii, 15, 19 n.1, 22–30, 45–47
 patient-researchers 27–30
 terminology xv
Peele, P. 44
pervasive developmental disorder not otherwise specified (PDD-NOS) 40, 45–47 *see also* autistic spectrum disorder

Pfizer 19 n.1
pharmaceutical industry xiii, 13–20, 33, 59
Phillips, J. 11
Phillips, K. 35
phobia 8–10, 29
Pinborough-Zimmerman, J. 43–44
Pincus, H. 47
post-traumatic stress disorder xii
premenstrual dysphoric disorder xiii, 6, 12
prevalence rates 26, 41–44, 47
promiscuous realism 60
Psychiatric News xii
psychoanalysis 2, 44, 49
Pulli, K. 37

Ramsay, J. xii
rapid eye movement sleep behavioural disorder 6
Reed, G. 58–59
Regier, D. xi, 1–2, 23, 42, 52, 55
reliability 26, 49–55
Research Agenda for DSM-V, A 1–3
Research Domain Criteria (RDoC) 57
restless legs syndrome 5
Rett's disorder 40
rubbish 36
Ruby, D. 39

schizophrenia 6, 52, 60
Schlaug, G. 37
service users *see* patients
sex offenders 8

sexual aversion disorder 10
sexual disorders 10
Shuer, L. 39
Siklos, S. 43
Singer, E. 45
skin picking *see* excoriation
sleep-wake disorders 10
social anxiety disorder 16
social (pragmatic) communication disorder 6, 42, 46
somatic symptom disorder 24
Spitzer, R. 27, 50–53
SSRI (selective serotonin re-uptake inhibitors) 28–29, 34
Strasser, S. 36
stuttering xii

Tierney, C. 41
Tourette's syndrome xii

trademark, DSM-5 26
transsexualism xii–xiii
trash 36

Verhoeff, B. 45, 55
Volkmar, F. 9–10, 42

Waite, R. xii
waste 36
Whoriskey, P. 14
Wieczner, J. 33
Wilkins, J. 40
Williams, J. 50, 52
Williams, K. 11, 41
World Health Organisation (WHO) x, 58

"yellow card" system 28
Young, A. xii